PHONE COACHING
IN DIALECTICAL BEHAVIOR THERAPY

Guilford DBT® Practice Series
Alan E. Fruzzetti, *Series Editor*

This series presents accessible, step-by-step guides to essential components of dialectical behavior therapy (DBT) practice. Delving deeply into different aspects of DBT implementation—phone coaching, validation, chain analysis, family interventions, and more—series volumes distill the latest clinical innovations and provide practical help based on sound DBT principles and good science.

Phone Coaching in Dialectical Behavior Therapy
Alexander L. Chapman

Chain Analysis in Dialectical Behavior Therapy
Shireen L. Rizvi

Phone Coaching in Dialectical Behavior Therapy

Alexander L. Chapman

Series Editor's Note by Alan E. Fruzzetti

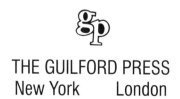

THE GUILFORD PRESS
New York   London

Library of Congress Cataloging-in-Publication Data
Names: Chapman, Alexander L. (Alexander Lawrence) author.
Title: Phone coaching in dialectical behavior therapy / Alexander L. Chapman.
Description: New York : The Guilford Press, [2019] | Series: Guilford
    dbt[registered mark] practice series | Includes bibliographical references
    and index.
Identifiers: LCCN 2018015006| ISBN 9781462537358 (paperback) |
    ISBN 9781462537365 (hardcover)
Subjects: LCSH: Dialectical behavior therapy. | BISAC: MEDICAL / Psychiatry /
    General. | SOCIAL SCIENCE / Social Work. | PSYCHOLOGY / Emotions.
Classification: LCC RC489.B4 C434 2019 | DDC 616.89/142—dc23
LC record available at https://lccn.loc.gov/2018015006

About the Author

Alexander L. Chapman, PhD, RPsych, is Professor and Clinical Science Area Coordinator in the Department of Psychology at Simon Fraser University (SFU), in Burnaby, British Columbia, Canada, and president of the Dialectical Behavior Therapy (DBT) Centre of Vancouver. Dr. Chapman directs the Personality and Emotion Research Laboratory at SFU, where he studies the role of emotion regulation in borderline personality disorder, self-harm, impulsivity, and other behavioral problems. He has published numerous scientific articles, chapters, and books; presents widely at scientific conferences; and is on the editorial boards of *Personality Disorder: Theory, Research, and Treatment*; *Journal of Personality Disorders*; and *Behavior Therapy*. Dr. Chapman is a DBT Trainer and Consultant with Behavioral Tech, LLC. He regularly gives local, national, and international workshops and invited talks on DBT and the treatment of borderline personality disorder; has consulted with and trained clinicians in Canada, the United States, and the United Kingdom; and trains and supervises clinical psychology students. He is a recipient of awards including the Young Investigator's Award from the National Education Alliance for Borderline Personality Disorder, the Early Career Scientist Practitioner Award from the Canadian Psychological Association, and an 8-year Career Investigator Award from the Michael Smith Foundation for Health Research.

Seres Editor's Note

Dialectical Behavior Therpy—Then and Now

This new book series was developed to eet the increasing needs of practitioners to learn how to do dialecal behavior therapy (DBT®) well—in an adherent and competently. DBT was developed originally for suicidal and/or self-harming patis with borderline personality and related disorders. While the DBTeatment manual (Linehan, 1993a), the revised *DBT Skills Training Nual* (Linehan, 2015b), and the *DBT Skills Training Handouts and Wheets* (Linehan 2015a) provide therapists with the entire treatment)tocol, other aspects of the treatment—chain analysis, validation, ph coaching, family interventions, consultation team, and effective uf dialectical strategies, to name a few—have developed considerablyond the original treatment manual. It is for this reason that we develd this series, with the support of Dr. Marsha M. Linehan, to help prtioners enhance and refine their skills and deliver DBT to their patiemore effectively, according to present DBT standards and practices.

When the young psychologist Marslinehan and her colleagues at the University of Washington develope3T in the 1980s, it was not at all clear if the treatment would be suful, in terms of both treatment efficacy for people who are chroni suicidal and self-harming (typically referred to as having borderlinsonality disorder, or BPD), for whom the treatment was developed, a:ceptance and adoption for use by the therapeutic community, who lad struggled to treat people with these problems. In order to understand how the accessible guides in this series enhance the literature and promote adherence to current DBT principles and practices, we must first show how they fit into the overall structure of DBT treatment and the treatment context for BPD and related problems that have evolved over time.

Looking back 30 years or more, it is stunning to see the impact Dr. Linehan's work has had on the field. Before her work became widely disseminated and accepted, suicidal and/or self-harming people with BPD faced rampant stigmatization, sense of hopelessness about recovery, and a complete absence of empirically supported treatments. Needless to say, people with DBT faced a bleak prognosis. At the time, DBT was available only in a small clinic at the University of Washington. There was no treatment manual or skill manual; there were no clear ways to teach, disseminate, or implement the treatment effectively.

Where are we now? Stigma has been significantly reduced, hope has increased, there is a general recognition among professionals that BPD and related problems are treatable (although there is still a long way to go), and an impressive volume of studies evidence strong support for DBT's efficacy and effectiveness. There is a widely read treatment manual (Linehan, 1993a), and both an original (1993b) and enhanced and updated skills manual (15a, 2015b). Well-trained teams in outpatient, residential, hospital, and other settings treat thousands of people every day with DBT, not only across the United States but in dozens of countries and on every continent. Many of these treatment providers have demonstrated both their commitment and their abilities by becoming certified as DBT therapists, which requires rigorous demonstration of their skills as DBT providers. In addition, other effective treatments, generally also nonpejorative toward people with BPD and related difficulties, have been empirically established or are under development.

In addition, applications and adaptations of DBT have been successfully developed for a host of problems other than BPD per se (i.e., severe problems related to emotion regulation) and across a variety of treatment—and, more recently, prevention—settings. It's not a surprise that Dr. Linehan was just featured one of the 100 "Great Scientists" of all time ("Great Scientists," 2018).

DBT is an *integrative* treatment that includes a whole set of interventions (modes and functions of treatment). DBT includes not only individual therapy but also many other modalities that serve different functions in treatment, such as group skills training, telephone coaching, family interventions, and an ongoing consultation team. DBT integrates the techniques and scope of acceptance-oriented therapies (e.g., support, warmth, encouragement) with the strategies and precision of behavior therapies and emotion science (e.g., precise treatment targets, scientific analysis of behavior [emotions, thoughts, actions]) and focuses on psychological and social skills as *solutions* to a range of problems. Dozens of controlled studies support the effectiveness of DBT in creating safety, stability, and self-control while minimizing treatment dropout, as well as improving mood, self-esteem, relationships, family, school and job functioning, and so forth. Largely due to stable outcomes and reduced relapse, costs of DBT compared to alternative treatments are also significantly reduced in the long term.

The DBT Model

The treatment model views *emotion dysregulation* as the core of a variety of emotional, cognitive (thinking), relational, identity (self-concept), and behavioral problems. Emotion dysregulation increases or exacerbates behavioral dysregulation (out-of-control actions, including impulsivity), cognitive dysregulation (trouble thinking and problem solving), interpersonal dysregulation (difficulties in relationships), and self-dysregulation (problems with self-esteem, identity, negative self-views). Consequently, many common co-occurring problems (suicidal and nonsuicidal self-injury, depression, anxiety, eating disorders, posttraumatic stress disorder, substance abuse, aggression, problems in relationships, etc.) are similarly understood either as dysfunctional attempts to regulate emotion or as natural consequences of chronic emotion dysregulation. The overarching goal of DBT is to help people create lives worth living by helping them learn psychological and social skills to regulate, or manage, their emotions—earlier in treatment tolerating and re-regulating secondary emotions, and later in treatment identifying, accurately labeling, allowing, expressing accurately, and managing primary emotions. Much of the treatment is built around these principles.

Chronic and severe emotion dysregulation is hypothesized to result from an ongoing *transaction* between the person's emotion vulnerabilities and ongoing invalidation from others in the social and family environment, which often promotes self-invalidation as well. Emotion vulnerability is influenced by temperament, conditioning, and present biological disposition resulting from learning and current circumstances and manifests as emotional sensitivity and reactivity, along with often slow return to emotion equilibrium. Invalidating responses can take a variety of forms, from the obviously critical and emotionally abusive to well-meaning misunderstandings that occur because of temperamental differences, inaccurate expression, or miscommunication between people and their family members and others.

Five Core Functions of Comprehensive DBT

DBT consists of components or modes that address the five essential functions of treatment:

1. Help people learn new psychological, emotional, and social/relationship skills, typically via skills training groups.
2. Help people generalize those skills to their real, everyday lives, in situations that have elicited less skillful responses in the past, which includes detailed planning, *in vivo* coaching, and practicing skills in the "real" world.
3. Help people collaborate on their treatment targets and enhance their motivation to replace overlearned dysfunctional behaviors with more skillful alternatives, primarily through individual psychotherapy, and also in other ways, depending on treatment setting.
4. Help people manage their social and family relationships to build better relationships and elicit more support, understanding, and validation and help family members become more validating and supportive in return.
5. Provide ongoing support, validation, problem solving, and skill building for therapists to enhance their motivation and skills through regular team consultation meetings.

DBT Skills

Learning key psychological, emotional, and social skills is believed to be central in helping patients learn to regulate their emotions, build satisfying relationships, and thrive. These include skills to:

1. Increase attention control and nonjudgmental awareness and build a more positive self-concept or identity (mindfulness).

2. Understand emotions, increase positive emotions, decrease vulnerability to negative reactions, accept negative emotional experiences, and change negative emotional experiences (emotion regulation skills).

3. Build empathy and improve relationships while balancing assertion with self-respect (interpersonal skills).

4. Tolerate highly distressing experiences without doing things impulsively that increase dysregulation overall (distress tolerance skills).

5. Balance competing goals, interests, and perspectives and build cognitive and emotional flexibility (dialectics, or the middle path, along with "wise mind").

Over time, some additional skills have become part of the DBT lexicon, such as dialectical and validation skills for patients and their families, specific skills for people with substance use problems, and so on (cf. Fruzzetti, Payne, & Hoffman, in press; Miller, Rathus, & Linehan, 2007; Rathus & Miller, 2015).

Of course, principles of learning are at the core of any behavior therapy, including DBT. In particular, there are three overlapping phases of learning: (1) the acquisition phase, in which the basics of the skill are learned, typically in skills training groups designed to be optimal learning environments; (2) the strengthening phase, in which the person practices the skill, typically in planned ways, in groups or with the therapist or at home; and (3) the generalization phase, in which the person's skill has become robust enough that he or she can employ it when needed in his or her life, often spontaneously. Of course, in addition to the teaching/training and coaching that occur in skills training groups and in individual sessions, in outpatient settings *in vivo* coaching can help to generalize skills (mostly by text or telephone) and manage between-session problems.

Acceptance and Validation

Throughout DBT, treatment providers strive to understand and validate the primary emotional experience of their patients, along with other valid behaviors, and help clients validate themselves. We do not validate things that are not, in fact, valid. This is a complex task, learning to discriminate the valid aspects of any given behavior from the invalid ones. For example, certain impulsive and/or destructive behaviors (e.g., self-harm, substance use) are typically primary targets for change because they are invalid ways to solve problems or enhance quality of life in the long term. Yet, they are valid in the sense that they do often "work" to reduce, avoid, or escape painful negative emotional arousal. Understanding and validating what is valid, even in the most dysfunctional behavior, is a key therapeutic activity that helps the client feel understood (validated), increases motivation for change, builds the therapeutic relationship, and thus increases collaboration for change. Consequently, therapist validation not only has value in itself (feeling understood, cared about, etc.), it also helps regulate the person and promotes change.

Change, Problem Solving, and Behavior Therapy

Within a therapeutic context based on understanding, acceptance, and validation, the therapist targets dysfunctional behaviors for change, pushing patients to substitute skillful alternatives for the problematic reactions and dysfunctional behaviors for which they sought treatment. Utilizing a carefully constructed treatment target hierarchy, DBT therapists and the DBT team can employ all the components of learning and behavior therapy: (1) careful assessment, using chain analysis; (2) development of solutions on the chain and replacement of dysfunctional "links" in the chain that led to a dysfunctional or undesired behavior with a skillful alternative (this includes learning skills, noted above); (3) behavioral rehearsal and other commitment strategies to foster the difficult change process; and (4) all the techniques of behavior therapy to help the person actually use the skill when needed (e.g., stimulus control, reinforcement/contingency management, exposure and response prevention).

Dialectics

Balancing acceptance and validation with change, problem solving, and behavior therapy is complicated, and there are no algorithms to guide us because each context is unique. Rather, the therapist must balance these dialectically in the service of effectiveness. Every strategy in DBT has an "opposite" of equal value that must be considered and balanced in order to help people change in the ways they want to change. Just as acceptance and validation must be balanced with change and problem solving, intervening on behalf of clients is balanced by consulting with clients to empower them to intervene on their own behalf; communicating in a warm, genuine, and caring way must be balanced with irreverence, insistence, and matter-of-fact communication; and emotion must be balanced with reason (and vice versa).

Interventions in the Social and Family Environments

Although an important component of DBT from the beginning, social and family interventions are areas that have shown enormous growth and development since the first wave of DBT was developed and implemented. For example, fully developed applications of DBT have been shown to be effective with parents, couples, and families, and in school systems, and are being used to prevent the development of emotion dysregulation problems or to intervene early to help clients avoid full-blown problems related to emotion dysregulation. All of these efforts utilize the core principles of DBT, but of course have expanded the strategies and techniques to be effective in these new domains. Their growth and development are a positive testament to the coherence and effectiveness of DBT from the beginning.

What DBT Is and What It Is Not

Given the strong empirical foundation for DBT, it is no surprise that many clinicians want to offer DBT as part of their therapeutic toolbox. However, DBT is complex and requires considerable time, effort, and dedication to learn well. So, it is also not surprising that a wide range of treatments are offered under the DBT "label," but are of varying DBT quality. This is confusing for consumers at best, and of course fraudulent at worst. Imagine if a surgeon thought, "I've never had the training to do this procedure, but I read a little bit about it, so I can advertise myself as an expert in it." No one would want this surgeon performing a procedure on them. Fortunately, a certification process for DBT therapists, and their DBT teams, is now underway. This is a significant positive development both for people who need treatment (they will know what they are getting) and for DBT therapists (they will have objective measures that show they are doing excellent work).

How This Book Series Fits into the Development of DBT

DBT is, at least metaphorically, a living, breathing, and always growing and evolving treatment. It expands and changes in a dialectical manner. We use the therapy according to the model (the "thesis" or "proposition"); when something is not working well, DBT therapists innovate within the treatment ("antithesis" in which we employ theory and science to develop something new). In response to data and research findings about these innovations, we find some things work and others do not; ultimately, some new strategies or interventions become established and integrated with the old (synthesis, now established treatment), and stay that way until a situation arises in which they do not work well, and then further innovation (further antitheses) is engaged.

The original text (Linehan, 1993a) remains relevant and wise and includes an enormous amount of thoughtful and effective guidance. DBT has evolved since 1993 to include many more things (applications in new settings, extensions of principles and strategies, new skills, etc.) that could not have been anticipated at the time the book was written. This book series presents DBT as it is today, synthesizing the old and the new, built on the original treatment manual.

For example, the current (and first!) book to be published in this series focuses on telephone consultation with clients/patients. This idea of coaching suicidal and self-harming clients by telephone between sessions was an innovative notion and was greeted by many therapists as a potentially frightening aspect of treatment. Were clients going to abuse their phone privileges, intrude on therapists' lives, and make neverending demands on therapists' time? This book shows how to observe therapeutic limits, coach but not provide treatment, and use phone time to effectively advance treatment. We have learned a lot about the nuances of skill coaching on the telephone, how things might be different for teens than they are for adults, and other aspects of phone coaching that only emerged over time with a lot of effort, innovation, and empirical evaluation. At its heart, phone coaching is an evidence-based method of helping people generalize new skills they have learned to situations in their life as they unfold in real time. Consequently, this book is not only essential for outpatient DBT therapists and teams, but is also potentially useful for any therapist, coach, or even parent whose role includes helping another person use new skills in difficult situations, in particular in situations of escalating negative emotional arousal.

Dr. Alexander Chapman is a former postdoctoral fellow of Dr. Linehan's and an expert in DBT as a researcher, clinician, trainer, and supervisor, having worked in and headed up outpatient programs for many years. Given his wealth of experience, it is not surprising that this small book packs in enormous wisdom about the principles of phone coaching, as well as many nuances that help the person doing the coaching find that effective dialectical balance, integrating or synthesizing understanding, acceptance, and validation with a strong push for generalized learning in the moment. Any new skill can be a challenge to learn, even in a supportive therapeutic environment. When clients need to apply skills in real time, they can become easily demoralized, especially when they are under duress, stuck in a challenging situation, or in the midst of a full-blown suicidal state. Any of us could become "deskilled" under any of these conditions. This book shows how to help effectively in the direst of circumstances. Dr. Chapman provides the reader with both the foundational principles that form the basis of any DBT intervention, along with highly practical tips, examples, transcripts, and suggestions for effective implementation of phone coaching.

Moreover, Dr. Chapman walks through a variety of coaching situations, including dangerous ones that include patient urges to self-harm or commit suicide. He shows how coaching from the therapist can eventually be transformed into further empowering clients by teaching them how to use the skills themselves. Nuances of the therapists' approach—how they balance the acceptance/change dialectic—are conveyed in helpful ways that are sure to provide maximum effectiveness for the client without burning out the therapist. Indeed, Dr. Chapman consistently provides a realistic view of what is likely to be helpful for clients and *does not* promote therapist burnout at the same time. In DBT, preventing burnout and maintaining job satisfaction is an essential function of the treatment that must be met: a burned-out therapist won't provide after-hours telephone coaching at all, and this would deprive clients of important help, guidance, and learning opportunities.

Throughout this manual, Dr. Chapman manages to dispel myths, provide encouragement, and offer empirical evidence for various strategies, while constantly weaving in practical guidelines for what to do under different circumstances, as well as what principles support which techniques. This book is a terrific first book in our series precisely because it takes an essential component of the larger treatment and delves deeply into its implementation, providing practical help built on both sound principles and good science. Like this book, the entire series intends to augment, rather than replace, the current DBT manuals (Linehan, 1993a, 2015a, 2015b). Each book will illustrate many new developments, guided by both clinical innovation and sound research, that constitute DBT today.

ALAN E. FRUZZETTI, PhD

References

Fruzzetti, A. E., Payne, L., & Hoffman, P. D. (in press). Dialectical behavior therapy with families. In L. A. Dimeff, K. Koerner, & S. Rizvi (Eds.), *Dialectical behavior therapy in clinical practice: Applications across disorders and settings* (2nd ed.). New York: Guilford Press.

Great scientists: The geniuses and visionaries who transformed our world. (2018). *Time (Special Edition)*. New York: Time, Inc.

Linehan, M. M. (1993a). *Cognitive-behavioral treatment of borderline personality disorder*. New York: Guilford Press.

Linehan, M. M. (1993b). *Skills training manual for treating borderline personality disorder*. New York: Guilford Press.

Linehan, M. M. (2015a). *DBT skills training handouts and worksheets* (2nd ed.). New York: Guilford Press.

Linehan, M. M. (2015b). *DBT skills training manual* (2nd ed.). New York: Guilford Press.

Miller, A. L., & Rathus, J. H., & Linehan, M. M. (2007). *Dialectical behavior therapy with suicidal adolescents*. New York: Guilford Press.

Rathus, J. H., & Miller, A. L. (2015). *DBT skills manual for adolescents*. New York: Guilford Press.

Contents

CHAPTER 1

Introduction and Overview

When I first bring up phone coaching during talks or workshops, many audience members get that shocked deer-in-the-headlights look, as if I have just suggested that they should ask their clients to move in with them. Yet phone coaching is an important aspect of treatment, and can be managed in a way that doesn't end up by turning clients into roommates. In this book, I focus on why we do it, how to make it effective, and ways to avoid common pitfalls. I am excited to have the opportunity to put what I have learned about phone coaching in dialectical behavior therapy (DBT®) on paper, and to give clinicians clear principles and practical guidance on how to approach this aspect of treatment.

As anxiety-provoking as phone coaching can be, it is an integral part of treatment. DBT clinicians share a common goal: to ensure that our clients receive full, comprehensive DBT (including individual therapy, group skills training, and phone coaching). And this unfortunately requires them to be available to their clients in between sessions, largely during their personal time. Even therapists who have read the original DBT manual (Linehan, 1993a), which only included under 10 pages on the topic, might find themselves ill-equipped and reluctant to navigate phone coaching. Moreover, many clinicians wonder (and worry about) how phone coaching works in a practical sense. How many calls can you expect to receive? How many is it reasonable for you to be willing to receive? Do you truly need to be available 24 hours a day, 7 days a week? How do you get off the phone with clients who won't hang up? What do

1

you do when a client calls too often? How can you manage suicide risk during a brief phone call? This book will help answer all these practical questions and more.

In this first chapter, I provide a brief overview of phone coaching in DBT. I begin by discussing whom this book is for and what phone coaching is and is not. I also describe the primary reasons for and functions of phone coaching in DBT. Subsequently in this section, I discuss common concerns and dispel myths about phone coaching. Finally, I will provide some guidance on how to navigate the rest of this book.

Who Can Gain from Reading This Book

This book is addressed to mental health clinicians, students, or other professionals who would like to incorporate phone coaching into their practice. Although the focus is on phone coaching as it is conducted in DBT, I have tried to make these principles relevant to a range of clinical populations and professionals trained in other treatment modalities. You do not need to be a well-trained DBT clinician to start to make use of these principles and strategies right away.

If you have not received any significant DBT training or primarily provide cognitive-behavioral therapy (CBT) or other treatments, the material in this book may help you to enhance your practice in many ways. The establishment of new, effective coping strategies is a common benefit of CBT and other approaches. For new coping strategies to make a difference in clients' lives, however, clients need to use and practice them in everyday situations. Phone coaching is designed to help clients do just that. Regardless of your treatment approach, therefore, the principles and strategies in this book will give you new ways to help clients learn and apply effective coping skills to learn more about themselves, manage stress, improve relationships, and achieve their important goals. Moreover, as phone coaching was developed in the treatment of complex patients (i.e., those with borderline personality disorder or who are highly suicidal), I believe the strategies discussed in this book can be useful for a range of clients, especially those whose emotion regulation (ER) problems play a role in their difficulties.

For those who are experienced DBT or CBT clinicians, the book offers practical guidance on how to conceptualize and implement phone coaching. I am a seasoned DBT and CBT clinician, and I have probably made most of the top 10 mistakes a clinician can make with phone coaching (and there actually is a list of such mistakes; see Manning, 2011). In fact, I could have used a book like this one much earlier in my own career, and I probably couldn't have written it without learning from my many mistakes! Finally, I believe this book could be useful for practitioners who may only rarely use phone coaching but would like to incorporate more coaching and generalization strategies into their clinical work.

What Is Phone Coaching?

Phone coaching involves the clinician being available between sessions to guide the client in the use of skills learned in therapy. Although such coaching typically occurs over the phone, clinicians increasingly have used other forms of communication, such as e-mail, texts or other instant messaging (e.g., What's app?), or video-calling platforms, such as Skype, FaceTime, or others. With the advent of e-therapy, therapists increasingly use various messaging mechanisms (often built into apps or through secure Web interfaces) to coach and guide clients through various therapy modules. Throughout this book, I continue to refer to all of these forms of between-session communications as "phone coaching," but at times I discuss specific issues pertaining to electronic communication methods.

The primary goal of phone coaching is to guide clients to use skills effectively in their natural environments. Clients might, for example, call the clinician when they are particularly upset about an interpersonal conflict and unsure how to cope effectively with their emotional reactions. In those instances, the clinician provides the client with suggestions on relevant skills and how to use them to deal with his or her specific situation.

Although the primary goal of phone coaching is to remind clients how to best use their skills, there are other key topics that can be addressed over the phone. Sometimes clients want to address relationship issues that have arisen in a previous session. The client might, for example, call the clinician if he is upset about an interaction that occurred in the therapy session and believes the issue can't wait until the next session. For instance, if the client felt hurt or angry in response to something that the clinician did or said, and delaying the discussion might lead to other problems (e.g., the client avoiding the next session or arriving in an emotionally dysregulated state), then talking this through might avert adverse consequences.

Another common reason for clients to call is that they are experiencing an emergency or crisis. When this occurs, clinicians help clients use skills to manage or reduce the crisis or avoid making it worse (e.g., by engaging in harmful behaviors), as described in Chapter 7. Although suicide crisis calls regularly occur in DBT, most DBT clinicians encourage their clients to call long before crises occur.

In less frequent instances, clients may call to report on progress, provide updates about critical or important issues, or discuss other less pressing matters. Finally, sometimes clinicians themselves might use phone coaching in creative ways to enhance progress. A clinician might, for example, use scheduled phone coaching calls to help a depressed client get out of bed or to encourage a client to use skills to make it to her therapy session. In other cases, a therapist might use phone coaching as a form of contingency management to reinforce progress. A client, for example, might be allowed to call the therapist only when he has made progress or engaged in specific, agreed-upon behaviors, such as the practice of a specific skill or the completion of a particular task like submitting a job application.

What Is Phone Coaching Not?

Phone coaching is not therapy over the phone. Imagine that you are a coach for a hockey team (some readers are going to have to put up with the fact that the author is Canadian). Coaching on the fly, during the game, is akin to phone coaching in DBT. Given that the game is so fast-paced and the stakes are so high and that intense coaching focus and rapid-fire decisions are required, you must efficiently convey your message to the players during the couple of minutes when they're on the bench. You also might need to call out directives or make suggestions while the players are actually on the ice. Your statements need to be clear, succinct, direct, and to the point. You also need to focus on the present and the near- or short-term future (e.g., the next 5 minutes of the game). This would not be the time for intense analysis of the players on the other team, how your own players can improve their game over time, thoughts and feelings about their performance, how to improve fitness, prepare for the playoffs, and so on.

Similarly, phone coaching involves efficient coaching when the client is in the middle of the game, living his everyday life and navigating

challenging situations. As such, phone coaching tends to be brief, directive, present-focused, to the point, and efficient. A phone coaching call is
not the venue in which to solve the client's relationship problems, school
or employment difficulties, depression, or other challenges that require
consistent therapeutic work over time. The focus is on the here-and-now
and typically on what the client can do now and in the near future to
regulate or tolerate his or her emotions.

Coaching also is not crisis management or suicide prevention. Phone
coaching in DBT is often mistaken for a crisis call or suicide prevention
service. As I discuss in Chapter 3, which focuses on orienting the client
to phone coaching, it is important for the clinician to clarify that the
primary purpose of phone coaching is to generalize skills from therapy to
the client's everyday life. The primary goal is not to prevent suicide, to
manage suicide risk, or to navigate emergencies. Although a client may
call in the midst of a suicidal crisis, the ideal goal is to help her reduce
suicide crisis calls over time and use phone coaching primarily to transfer
skills to everyday life.

Why Do We Use Phone Coaching?

There are several reasons to use phone coaching. The paramount reason
is to help the client generalize skills from therapy to the natural environment. When skills coaching occurs while the client is navigating real-
life situations, he can try out the skills right then. In typical outpatient
therapy, the clinician spends only 1 to 2 hours per week and sometimes
even less time with the client. Therapy typically takes place in a setting
that is markedly different from the client's everyday life. Even the therapy
relationship differs dramatically from the client's relationships with family, friends, partners, or colleagues. It's not always clear whether the client
can use skills learned in the therapy context in everyday life when she or
he needs them most. Phone coaching, therefore, is one of a variety of generalization strategies (some of which are discussed in Chapter 9) geared
toward helping the client transfer skills from the therapeutic setting into
relevant everyday-life situations. Phone coaching should not be the only
generalization strategy used in the treatment of complex clients. Rather,
I recommend that clinicians embed phone coaching within a broader set
of generalization strategies. Over time, of course, it is useful to help the
client learn to guide him- or herself in the use of skills. In Chapter 9, I

discuss a broader set of generalization strategies as well as ways to help the client develop self-coaching skills.

Another potential benefit of phone coaching is that a well-timed phone coaching call may prevent short-term problems and help clients avoid compounding already stressful situations. When we teach clients distress tolerance skills in DBT, we often emphasize the notion that some of these skills (crisis survival strategies; Linehan, 2015) help the client to avoid making a difficult situation worse. Phone coaching can work in the same way. The client experiencing emotional distress following an interpersonal conflict, for example, might receive the suggestions, encouragement, and motivation she needs to avoid behaviors that might further inflame the situation. I have had many phone coaching calls with clients experiencing urges to engage in actions that would make their situations worse, such as self-injury, angry outbursts, revenge seeking, stalking, drug use, and so on. Particularly for clients in the first stage of DBT ("stage one"; Linehan, 1993a), impulse control and self-regulation are not well-developed skills. These clients, therefore, may need a little extra help and support from a clinician who knows the skills and can help encourage and motivate them to use the skills. Although it may sound like this benefit of phone coaching is akin to simply putting out fires in the client's life, some fires must be extinguished in order to avoid disastrous long-term consequences (e.g., suicide). Individual therapy sessions are there to help clients learn how to avoid starting these fires in the first place.

A third key benefit of phone coaching is the sense of support and connection that the client often feels when a caring and helpful clinician is available for assistance. Although this book is meant to be broadly applicable across many clinical populations, I will make a brief point here about treating people with borderline personality disorder (BPD) and related complex mental health problems. Marsha M. Linehan (1993a) has described people with BPD as the "ultimate outsiders." They often feel alienated, afraid, and drawn to interpersonal connection all at once. The biosocial theory underlying DBT suggests that invalidating environments in which the individual did not receive adequate care, support, or guidance in understanding and managing emotions contribute to the development of BPD (Crowell, Beauchaine, & Linehan, 2009; Linehan, 1993a). Indeed, people with BPD often have serious interpersonal dysfunction that persists for many years (Choi-Kain, Zanarini, Frankenberg, Fitzmaurice, & Reich, 2010). Establishing an effective, caring, and supportive relationship with a clinician who is willing to help in the client's everyday life may decrease interpersonal conflict and alienation. Interestingly, theories of suicide historically have emphasized the role of alienation and social disconnection in suicidal thoughts and behaviors (e.g., "egoistic suicide"—Durkheim, 1897; "thwarted belongingness"—Joiner, 2005). While phone coaching is not a suicide prevention service, and it would be naïve to think that we can prevent suicide, this mode of intervention (perhaps more so than many others) may help to address clients' feelings of disconnection or alienation.

Finally, another benefit of phone coaching is that it can give the client the opportunity to learn how to ask for help effectively (Linehan, 1993a). Effectively asking for help can be considered a skill, and some clients (and probably many clinicians) could use help with this skill. Some clients ask for help in a demanding, aggressive manner; others ask for a tremendous amount of help without considering the effect of this help seeking on their social supports; others never ask for help and consequently don't get the support they need. Still others become hurt and angry when others don't provide the support they need but never asked for. Phone coaching is an excellent training ground for clients to learn to effectively seek help and support. To ensure that clients receive effective training, the clinician should notice and comment on effective and ineffective help-seeking behaviors, and regularly debrief phone coaching calls during individual therapy sessions (discussed in Chapter 3 on structuring phone coaching calls).

Common Concerns and Myths

Many clinicians fear how phone coaching will affect their personal lives. Many assume that emotionally dysregulated clients will "bother" them at all hours of the day and night. They fear that their availability by phone will set a problematic precedent, blurring the boundaries of the therapy relationship and fostering dependency on the part of the client. Now that DBT has been disseminated broadly, most clinicians are already aware of and willing to use phone coaching. That said, several myths about this intervention persist. Below, I explore common clinical concerns, many of which turn out to be unfounded. I am also hoping that, throughout this book, you will learn that phone coaching can be a powerful and manageable intervention.

Phone Coaching Will Lead to Stress and Burnout

Perhaps the most common concern about phone consultation is that the clinician will be overwhelmed with calls, and suffer from stress and professional burnout. Fortunately, many of us who have been doing DBT for a long time have discovered that we are rarely in this situation. Anecdotally, among the DBT clinicians that I know, most of us have had only a few DBT clients with whom we have approached burnout in relation to phone coaching. The vast majority of clients do not even call. In fact, I have had to encourage reluctant clients to call far more often than I have confronted clients who were calling too much. Those who do call tend to use phone coaching appropriately and are grateful for the help. Over 90% of the time, I end phone coaching calls feeling good about the call and satisfied that I have helped my client.

Although few studies have addressed the topic, findings suggest that clinicians should be able to incorporate phone coaching into their work with minimal risk of burnout. In one study of complex clients with eating disorders receiving 13 weeks of DBT, less than half (47.2%) of the clients made use of phone coaching, only 3% of all calls lasted 20 minutes or longer, the average duration of calls was approximately 6 minutes, and the average number of calls was less than five (Limbrunner, Ben-Porath, & Wisniewski, 2011). In this study, 54% of calls occurred on the weekend, and 67% were between 4:00 and 11:00 P.M. In another study of 51 adults with BPD who attended 6 months of DBT, the average number of phone coaching contacts per month per client was 2.55 (Oliveira & Rizvi, in press). The highest utilizers of phone coaching ($n = 4$ participants, or 11% of the sample), accounting for 56% of all calls, made 79–143 calls over the 6-month period (Oliveira & Rizvi, in press). These data are consistent with the clinical experiences of many DBT clinicians. Infrequent, brief calls are the norm, mitigating the risk of clinician burnout. Furthermore, there is some evidence that phone calls with clients may reduce suicide attempts (Vaiva et al., 2006).

Clinicians Must Be Available at All Times

Another assumption is that the clinician must be available 24 hours a day, which would exceed many clinicians' personal and professional limits. In her original DBT manual, Linehan stated her belief that suicidal patients "must be told that they can call their therapists at any time—night or day, work days or holidays if necessary" (1993a, p. 503).

As we say in DBT, there is a dialectic here: On one hand, it is crucial to be available to highly suicidal clients, and, on the other hand, 24-hour availability can intrude in clinicians' lives; thus, some clinicians would choose not to do phone coaching if they had to be this available. As discussed further in Chapters 3 ("Orientation to Phone Coaching") and 8 ("Principles and Strategies to Address Challenges in Phone Coaching"), it is both important to be as available as possible and to observe limits and address therapy-interfering behavior (i.e., clients calling too much or during undesirable times) as it occurs. In many places where DBT is practiced, clinicians are permitted to have and observe their own limits around phone coaching. In our DBT team, for example, we accept clinicians' individual (and sometimes idiosyncratic) limits but emphasize that the approach most consistent with DBT principles is not to set limits ahead of time but to observe them as needed (monitor whether the client's behavior is pushing your limits). We ask that clinicians avoid narrowly defined limits, and that they accurately communicate their preferences to their clients ahead of time.

I try to maintain and observe limits that will keep me motivated to sustain phone coaching over the long term. For example, I often tell my clients that they can call me at any time, but that I generally go to bed between 9:30 and 10:30 P.M. and awaken around 5:30 or 6:00 A.M. I tell clients that, although I'm willing to take calls in the night, they might have difficulty reaching me, as my phone might not be readily available. I also mention that if they do reach me, I likely won't be as helpful as I am during regular waking hours. In case clients can't reach me in the middle of the night, I help them devise plans to use skills (e.g., a crisis survival plan, using some of the DBT distress tolerance skills; Linehan, 2015) or access support (e.g., calling others in their support networks, contacting crisis lines) during that period. I also tell clients that I nearly never answer my phone when it rings; thus, they must leave a brief message describing the kind of help they need, and I'll call them back when I'm available. I tell them that I prefer brief voice messages, and that I don't want them to leave messages reporting suicidal thoughts or urges. I also let them know I will sometimes get back to them quickly and sometimes several hours later. Normally, I say that I'll at least get back to them before I retire for the evening (I got this from Linehan's example; Linehan, 1993a), but that, at times, I may not be able to get back to them until the next morning. On my voicemail message, I state that I'll do my best to return calls within 24 hours. I also mention that clients experiencing a clinical emergency who can't wait for my call should access emergency services, contact a crisis line or their family physician, or visit the emergency room, and so forth.

Other colleagues navigate phone coaching differently. Some are available 24/7, whereas others are available only between 8:00 A.M. and 6:00 P.M. Still others answer their phones right away. Some of my colleagues prefer to receive a voice message or text indicating the seriousness or urgency (e.g., by the client texting 911) of the call, so they know how quickly to call back, and others want a detailed voice message describing the kind of help the client needs.

There are many ways to navigate phone coaching, and I encourage clinicians to consider their own limits, how phone coaching might affect their everyday lives, and to choose a method they can sustain. Phone coaching is, in some ways, analogous to incorporating some new self-care activity into your life, such as regular daily exercise. It's sometimes hard to find the time to do it, and if you take on more than you can sustain (e.g., deciding to get up at 4:00 A.M. and work-out for 3 hours every day), you're likely to burn out and quit. For self-care, I encourage people to only make changes they can feasibly keep up for more than a year. Similarly, clinicians who diligently observe limits around phone coaching will find themselves much more able to sustain this practice over the long run, compared with clinicians who fail to observe limits or those who set rigid limits up front and then become frustrated when their clients inevitably cross these limits. Many times, I've seen clinicians fail to observe limits and continue to take on more than they could sustain. This often results in burnout and urges to quit phone coaching entirely. Interestingly, clinicians in this situation often blame the client for calling (or texting/e-mailing) too much, when the clinician could have prevented this problem early on by observing limits consistently and seeking consultation and support from colleagues.

Phone Coaching Leads to Boundary Violations

Another common concern is that phone coaching invites boundary violations. Most mental health professionals are taught to avoid problematic multiple relationships or boundary violations, and some clinicians are vigilant regarding these issues. As such, clinicians sometimes believe that communication with clients during personal time changes the professional relationship into a more personal one. Instead of maintaining all therapeutic contact within the confines of a professional setting (or during professional working hours), the clinician is allowing the client to call (or text, e-mail, etc.) much like a friend would allow her to call for help or support. Clinicians might be concerned that the client will start viewing or treating them as friends.

Interestingly, although generalization of skills is the primary goal of phone coaching, another reason Linehan included phone coaching in DBT was that she wished to ensure that the therapy relationship contained the same elements as a real, genuine relationship (Linehan, personal communication). In any close relationship, people can freely call, e-mail, or text one another for support and help. We expect that our friends or family will be unavailable sometimes, but not that they are only accessible during working hours! And yet, these limitations often are the rule in therapy and can sometimes seem artificial or unnecessary to clients. Effective DBT phone coaching, therefore, involves balancing the qualities of genuineness and caring with principles, elements, and procedures promoting an ethical and professional therapy relationship.

Chapter 3, which focuses on orienting clients and observing limits, will provide guidance on how to set the therapeutic frame with respect to phone coaching. Problematic multiple relationship issues can often be avoided with adequate orientation to the roles of the clinician and the client and the procedures and expectations of phone coaching. Observing therapeutic limits consistently also can help the client and clinician catch and solve relationship issues related to phone coaching before these issues harm therapy.

Phone Coaching Will Encourage Clients to Be Dependent

Clinicians are understandably concerned that phone coaching will foster client dependency. The client might learn to call the clinician instead of use his or her own coping skills to manage difficult situations, which could possibly lead to an unhealthy dependency. In fact, some clients do indeed become dependent on phone coaching. I had a client who called me several times per week and always seemed to feel better following our calls. He thanked me profusely for my help, and I found the whole experience very gratifying. I thought I was doing good work and furthering the therapy by helping him through phone coaching. In reality, his frequent calls stretched my personal limits. The first clue to my rising resentment was a mild feeling of dread when I noticed his number on the call display.

I also noticed that the calls were not decreasing over time (which I might expect to see as therapy skills increasingly generalize to the client's life). I brought this issue up in our session, highlighted the effect of the phone calls on me, and discussed how they were working for the client. In doing so, we both discovered that phone coaching had become the client's primary method for regulating his emotions. Calling me had become the client's go-to skill. Once we discovered that, we knew exactly what needed to happen. We gradually reduced the frequency of the phone calls while helping him figure out how to use other skills to tolerate distress and regulate difficult emotions. Therefore, even if signs suggest that a client is becoming dependent on phone coaching, this dependency can usually be managed effectively in the context of an open, collaborative therapy relationship.

Dialectical Theory Applied to Phone Coaching

Because DBT is a *dialectical* treatment approach, dialectical principles influence how clinicians navigate phone coaching in DBT. Dialectical theory holds that reality consists of polar opposites, such as thesis versus antithesis, positive versus negative charge, matter versus antimatter, and so on. In DBT, the polar opposites are acceptance and change. In developing treatment for highly suicidal, complex clients, Linehan realized that a purely change-oriented approach, consisting of cognitive and behavioral interventions, was untenable, as clients experienced this approach as invalidating. The message was that all they needed to do to overcome a lifetime of intense suffering was to change their thoughts and behaviors and learn new coping skills. Change alone was inadequate. Acceptance alone, consisting of validation, empathetic listening, responsivity, warmth, and so forth, also was fundamentally invalidating and inadequate, as suicidal clients experiencing intense misery need their lives to change. To attain lives worth living, clients need to accept themselves, their thoughts, their emotions, and their experiences, and then they need to solve their problems and change their lives. To help complex clients, clinicians need to accept their clients the way they are and to help them improve and change in ways that bring them closer to their goals.

The dialectical framework of DBT reminds clinicians to seek a balance or synthesis of acceptance and change. Across modes of DBT, the central dialectic is that of validation versus problem solving. In phone coaching more specifically, the clinician seeks to balance validation of the client's experiences with problem solving in the form of skills coaching, which arguably solves the problem of the client's difficulty using skills when needed. Because of the brevity of phone coaching, the balance tends to weigh more heavily on the side of problem solving (skills coaching) than validation.

The clinician also should seek to balance the skills emphasized during phone coaching calls. Some of the DBT skills are more acceptance-oriented, such as mindfulness and some of the distress tolerance skills, whereas others are more change-oriented, such as interpersonal effectiveness and most of the ER skills. One of my clients, for example, recently presented with great difficulty tolerating boredom. He periodically felt keyed up, agitated, confused, and had difficulty concentrating, and when this happened, he began to have urges to engage in impulsive behavior, such as overspending. I believe I did an excellent job of coaching the client in skills to combat boredom, brainstorming stimulating activities, and encouraging the client to use distraction and opposite action. What was missing, however, were skills to accept and tolerate the experiences that accompanied boredom. Sometimes, life is boring, and there's value in learning how to experience boredom without having to avoid or escape it. Indeed, his urges to overspend could be considered a "symptom" of the broader problem of difficulty tolerating and accepting aversive inner experiences. Therefore, it's helpful for clinicians to remain attentive to their emphasis on acceptance versus change-oriented skills during phone coaching and to try to strike a balance that works well in view of each client's unique circumstances.

Another dialectical principle that I find especially helpful during phone coaching is that of working for synthesis. In phone coaching, the clinician and client will, at times, become polarized. The clinician might strongly urge the client to use skills and not to attempt suicide or self-injury, and the client might firmly insist that the skills won't work, and that she should harm herself. Whenever I become polarized in this or other scenarios, I remember a story from back when I was learning couples therapy in graduate school. My supervisor used to ask the couple to remember the last time they were in a heated conflict and to consider what their primary goal was in the heat of the moment. Most commonly, partners would say that their goal was to win the argument. Oddly enough, I never heard them say that their goal was to bring the relationship to a new, exciting level of intimacy. In any case, once the partners said that their goal was to win the argument, my supervisor would ask them, "What's the best possible outcome if you win the argument?" and then tell them that the best outcome was that "You're now married to the loser!"

Remembering this story and the dialectical strategy of working for synthesis, when I become polarized with clients during phone coaching, I try to remember to search for the wisdom or kernel of truth in the client's perspective and find a way to bring both of our perspectives together. A client, for example, once insisted that distress tolerance skills wouldn't fix her problems and are just superficial solutions at best. She said she spends most of her time trying to tolerate distress already. Meanwhile, I was urging her to use distraction and self-soothing (key distress tolerance skills) to get through a breakup without acting on urges to self-injure or making the situation worse by stalking the ex-girlfriend. She was refusing to use skills to "simply tolerate" her emotions, and I was insisting that she needs to tolerate for a period before we can do anything to improve the situation. We weren't getting anywhere. I had to step back, try to understand where she was coming from, and determine why she didn't want to use distress tolerance skills before we could move on. I asked her what was really making her not want to use these skills, and she told me she felt like she was out of gas, that she couldn't keep simply treading water and tolerating her feelings, and that she felt incredibly lonely and desperately wanted to reach out to her ex-girlfriend. Both of our positions were valid. She needed to ride out her self-injury urges and avoid making the situation worse by stalking her ex-girlfriend (my position) *and* was unlikely to find continued distraction successful and probably needed more support. Once we brought both of our positions together, we were able to come up with a plan that worked to get her through the evening. Working for synthesis, therefore, often involves bringing together the true or wise aspects of each person's position. A common way to do this in DBT is to use "both . . . and . . . " statements. Some examples are listed below:

- "It is *both* true that it is ridiculous for me to ask you to take suicide off the table when having an exit door makes life more tolerable *and* that if you stay camped out at the exit door, you won't be able to benefit from therapy and build a life worth living."

- "It's *both* true that you need a lot more support and more phone calls this week, *and* that I can't have any more calls with you without becoming burned-out and ineffective."

- "It's *both* true that self-injuring might take away your pain more quickly and easily than the skills I have to offer, *and* that the skills still work and won't make things worse."
- "It's *both* true that we need to solve the problems making you miserable, *and* that those problems are too big and complicated to solve on the phone right now."

Throughout this book, I try to demonstrate a dialectical approach to phone coaching. Aside from dialectical theory, other theoretical perspectives and principles also are applicable to phone coaching, including theory and principles for skills training, emotions and ER, and others. These are discussed in subsequent chapters in this book.

Basic Rules and Procedures

It often has been said that there are only two fixed rules in standard DBT (Linehan, 1993a). The first rule is that clients who miss four consecutive sessions are out of therapy. Relatedly, clients are not out of therapy *until* they have missed four consecutive sessions. This is often referred to as the *four-miss rule* (Linehan, 1993a). This rule only pertains to phone coaching insofar as clients who are out of therapy are also out of phone coaching.

The second rule pertains specifically to phone coaching. This is called the *24-hour rule*: Clients are not to have between-session communication with their clinicians for a 24-hour period following an instance of self-injury or a suicide attempt. The rationale for this rule is that the availability of the clinician in the time closely following an act of self-injury or a suicide attempt might inadvertently reinforce these behaviors. Contemporary models of self-injury and suicidal behavior underscore the importance of avoiding such reinforcement. For example, Nock's four-function model of self-injury posits that positive or negative social reinforcement sometimes maintains self-injury (Nock & Prinstein, 2004). In a recent daily-diary study, 60 recurrent self-injurers monitored their emotions, thoughts, social support, urges and thoughts about self-injury, and acts of self-injury over a 14-day period. Among those self-injurers who reported that someone else was aware of their self-injury, social support following self-injury predicted engagement in self-injury the following day (Turner, Cobb, Gratz, & Chapman, 2016). Clinicians providing support soon after self-injury might believe they're helping, but this kind of support might predict increased risk of self-injury.

In the therapeutic context, positive social reinforcement can include attention, warmth, validation, time spent interacting with the client, and other actions on the part of the clinician that occur contingent upon the client's engagement in self-injury. Negative social reinforcement might involve the withdrawal of demands or requests, the avoidance of distressing problem discussions, among other consequences contingent on the occurrence or report of self-injury. Social reinforcement, however, is probably not relevant to all clients who engage in self-injury or suicide attempts. For some clients, contact with the clinician immediately following self-injury might be aversive. One of my previous clients, for example, vehemently complained about the 24-hour rule for several months following the beginning of therapy. This client had a difficult time calling me and found the process of phone coaching to be incredibly embarrassing and anxiety-provoking. She also felt ashamed to ask for help. For her, talking to me immediately following self-injury might have been more likely to be punishment than reinforcement. My client almost convinced me to abandon or change the 24-hour rule, but when I finally said I was open to changing things, she said she would be more comfortable with me sticking to the treatment as it's supposed to be done! I'm glad I stuck to the 24-hour rule, as I think it's critical to eliminate the possibility, however remote, that I might exacerbate a client's self-injury. Notwithstanding, as DBT is a principal-driven rather than a rule-driven treatment, there may be times when the clinician chooses to abandon the 24-hour rule. Given the high-stakes and potential danger of reinforcing suicidal or self-injurious behavior, the clinician considering this should have a strong rationale for her or his decisions, based on a solid case formulation and ideally some evidence of the factors reinforcing or punishing the client's behavior.

It is important to note that some have argued that the 24-hour rule is not appropriate for most adolescents (Miller, Rathus, & Linehan, 2007). Adolescents may be less able to manage the aftermath of suicidal or self-injurious behavior, accurately estimate their need for medical attention, or access emergency services (Steinberg, Steinberg, & Miller, 2011). Clinicians should consider whether to apply this rule or some adapted form of it with older adolescents who are more capable of managing their risk (Steinberg et al., 2011). The key principle underlying the 24-hour rule is that it is critical to avoid reinforcing self-injury and suicidal behavior;

clinicians always should incorporate this principle (if not the rule per se) into their approach to phone coaching. If a clinician is available shortly after an episode of self-injury or suicidal behavior, he or she should ensure that the client does not receive any potentially reinforcing consequences that she does not receive when she has not recently self-injured or attempted suicide. The clinician might, for example, avoid being more warm or responsive than usual, dial-down reassuring or validating statements, get down to business quickly and spend less time than usual on the phone with the client, and so forth. The basic idea is that the clinician can take steps to avoid differentially reinforcing self-injurious or suicidal behavior even if he or she needs to talk to the client shortly after the behavior has occurred.

How the Book Is Organized

The first few chapters of this book discuss considerations to address when the clinician is either considering or starting to implement phone coaching. Effective phone coaching often requires preparation, including decisions regarding the use of phone coaching across the board, or only with specific clients; logistical issues and how phone coaching will fit within the clinician's practice setting; and limits to place on phone coaching. Clinicians using phone coaching also should consider whether they have a supportive network of peers or supervisors with whom to consult. These and other considerations are discussed in Chapter 2, which focuses on ways to set the stage for effective phone coaching.

I have often found that challenges with students, supervisees, and clients regularly stem from inadequate orientation. When the client is well oriented to the purpose, structure, and expectations of phone coaching, this mode of treatment often precedes smoothly and effectively. The focus of Chapter 3 is on the orientation of the client to the purposes and practicalities of phone coaching.

Phone coaching is also most effective when it is structured appropriately. Given the brief nature of phone coaching, structure in this mode of treatment is perhaps even more important than it is in longer, standard therapy sessions. Structure can facilitate efficient work and often helps distressed clients to feel regulated and organized. Chapter 4, therefore, focuses on effective ways to structure and navigate the beginning, middle, and ending portions of phone coaching calls.

As the primary focus of phone coaching is on coaching the client in effective skill use, clinicians also must be familiar with key principles and practices of skills coaching. Chapter 5 focuses on principles of skills acquisition, strengthening, and generalization, as well as key strategies for effective skills coaching. These strategies are not unique to phone coaching and can be helpful during individual therapy, skills training, case management, and coaching in milieu settings.

Often, DBT phone coaching, partly because it is so brief, focuses primarily on helping clients use skills to effectively tolerate or regulate overwhelming emotions. There is not enough time for lengthy discussions of problem areas or long-standing problems. The focus is usually on emotions in the present moment and near future. As such, the clinician needs to know about key principles of ER. It is also useful to have some knowledge of ER and distress tolerance skills that are commonly used during phone coaching in DBT. In Chapter 6, I describe a practical ER framework to guide the clinicians' conceptualization and selection of skills. Subsequently, I provide some guidance on how to coach clients in some core DBT distress-tolerance and ER skills.

Although I recommend that clinicians deemphasize crises or emergencies as reasons to call, suicide crisis calls will occur from time to time. Indeed, this may be why some clinicians are reluctant to embark upon phone coaching: The worry is that they will not be able to adequately assess and manage risk and make critical decisions on the fly. Awareness of empirically based practical principles guiding suicide risk assessment and management can help guide effective decision making regarding suicide risk. As such, Chapter 7 focuses on principles and strategies for suicide crisis calls. Comprehensive books and resources on suicide risk assessment and management exist (Bongar, Shekykhani, Kugel, & Giannini, 2015; Maldonado & Garcia, 2016; Simon, 2012; Stolberg & Bongar, 2009). For the purposes of this book, in Chapter 7 I discuss key DBT principles and procedures guiding these calls.

If a clinician follows all of the guidelines in Chapters 2 through 7, phone coaching will likely proceed smoothly and effectively, with few bumps in the road. Inevitably, however, phone coaching involves challenges. Most clinicians will have a client who calls too often; becomes angry, critical, or defensive on the phone; refuses to use or talk about skills; repeatedly calls in suicidal crises; repeatedly e-mails or texts despite the clinician's limits on these behaviors; and so on. At the same time, clinicians also may interfere with phone coaching by inadequately orienting the client to their limits, failing to observe limits consistently, staying on the phone too long, inadequately addressing suicide risk, expressing judgmental thoughts, trying to do therapy on the phone, among many other possibilities. Chapter 8, therefore, addresses these and other common challenges in phone coaching. The beginning of the chapter focuses on general principles in the management of therapy-interfering behavior, and the remainder addresses specific strategies and approaches to particular problem areas, with an emphasis on observing therapeutic limits.

Skills coaching in DBT is much like coaching or teaching skills in soccer, music, or math. Usually, the student or trainee receives more help and guidance in the early phases and then develops increased independence and the capacity to learn on his or her own over time. In addition to generalizing skills to daily life, clients will learn to be their own coaches, providing themselves with guidance, encouragement, and instruction, as well as seeking additional external support when needed. In the final chapter (Chapter 9), the focus is primarily on ways to help the client generalize skills to life outside of the therapy session and to the period following the end of treatment. In addition, Chapter 9 includes strategies to help the client learn how to coach her- or himself in the effective use of skills.

Before we move on to Chapter 2, there is one more important point to remember: Certain chapters in this book are purposely thorough and comprehensive. You may read through Chapter 4 on structuring phone coaching and think that there is no way you can do all of these things within a brief call. You would probably be correct. Think of some of the chapters in this book as very thorough prototypes or blueprints of DBT phone coaching. How you put everything together will vary according to your own skills, background, and situation, and how you plan to use phone coaching in your setting with your clients. You can always go back, however, to the blueprint whenever you are wondering how things have gone awry or what to do differently.

CHAPTER 2

Setting the Stage for Effective Phone Coaching

T o increase the effectiveness of phone coaching, some preparation is in order. The chances that DBT-oriented phone coaching will be successful increase when the clinician is committed to this approach, prepared to navigate the logistics of phone coaching, and conducts phone coaching in a manner that is consistent with the core principles and strategies of DBT. This chapter focuses on ways to set the stage and prepare for effective phone coaching.

Committing to Phone Coaching

Phone coaching requires a significant commitment. The clinician is committing to squeeze time in for the client between other work and personal commitments, often during off hours or leisure time. The first step in making a significant commitment is to carefully consider what you're getting yourself into and whether you're willing to do it. When we hire new clinicians or practicum students, we attend to their willingness to use phone coaching with clients. Even those clinicians who have no initial concerns about phone coaching, considering how phone coaching might affect their daily lives before committing to it can reduce surprise or resentment later on when client calls begin to take time away from other activities.

Some clinicians work for an agency or within a DBT program in which phone coaching is mandatory. Others can decide themselves whether to incorporate phone coaching into their work. Even if you are required to use phone coaching, coming up with good reasons as to why phone coaching will enhance your clinical practice can increase your intrinsic motivation to use this therapeutic tool. People often do a better job and are less resentful of activities that they find meaningful, even if these activities are mandatory. Some helpful questions to consider include:

"Why would I consider or do phone coaching?"

"If phone coaching is mandatory, how do I think it might improve my practice?"

"What are the potential benefits of phone coaching to me or my clients?"

"How might phone coaching affect how I manage my personal time?"

"What are the potential downsides of phone coaching?"

"What are the reasons *not* to do phone coaching?"

The clinician who already is on a DBT team might consider having another team member do a "commitment session" with her. Some DBT consultation teams automatically set up commitment sessions with new team members. These sessions involve core DBT commitment strategies (outlined in Linehan, 1993a) to help the new team member make a firm commitment to the various expectations of a DBT consultation team. Some of these strategies are reflected in the questions above, such as examining pros and cons (potential benefits and downsides of phone coaching). In a commitment session, a therapist can guide the clinician through these types of questions and discuss various aspects of a commitment to phone coaching. Ideally, the clinician will emerge from this session with a stronger commitment to phone coaching or will make a reasonable decision not to do it (if that decision is up to the clinician).

Jane,[1] for example, had always wanted to learn DBT and jumped on board with phone coaching despite initial reluctance to take time away from her family on evenings or weekends. She previously had worked in

---

[1] All cases are based on real patients, but names and other identifying details have been changed to protect privacy.

community mental health centers with complex clients and always had a sense that 1 to 2 hours per week in a therapy office wasn't quite enough for these clients. Her clients kept saying that they could think clearly and cope well in therapy and in group, but that they completely fell apart when crises arose at home. She began to realize that the link between what was happening in the therapy office and clients' everyday lives was missing. As a result, she and her clients kept hitting roadblocks on the path to recovery, and her work became increasingly stressful. Despite concerns about how it might fit into her personal life, Jane saw phone coaching as a novel way to encourage quicker progress and to feel more effective as a clinician. Thinking this decision (to join a DBT team and do phone coaching) through, she came up with a sustainable plan for how often she would be available to her clients, what she would tell her family when she needed to take a client call, and how she would manage potential problems, such as by bringing these up with her team and seeking advice on how to observe therapeutic limits.

Phone Coaching as an Ancillary Tool for Clinicians Not Doing Standard DBT

If you're not doing standard DBT, phone coaching can still be a helpful ancillary treatment tool. Phone availability to clients between sessions has long been used as a tool in other forms of therapy. Many clinicians will ask clients to call them if they find themselves in a challenging situation. Phone calls can be used to help clients apply skills to whatever problem they may face. Depressed clients, for example, can benefit from coaching on how to solve an interpersonal problem, or to get started that day with activity scheduling. Phone coaching also can facilitate other therapy modalities that require a fair amount of homework outside of sessions, such as those requiring exposure therapy. Clients engaging in imaginal or *in vivo* exposure therapy can benefit from coaching or guidance on how to stick with the exposure protocol, select the most appropriate situations for *in vivo* exposure, and cope with the emotional aftermath of exposures, among other issues. Clients working on substance use issues may need help with skills to manage urges or cravings or navigate high-risk situations without drinking or using drugs. Phone coaching could be potentially useful across many clinical populations, but it is important to recognize that systematic research on treatments including phone coaching (outside of DBT) is rare. That said, phone coaching in DBT has been defined and systematized in a way that it hasn't been in other therapeutic modalities.

I highly recommend that clinicians base the decision of whether to use phone coaching with a client on a solid individual case formulation. In many therapy orientations, case formulations include the following elements: (1) relevant history, (2) presenting problems or concerns, (3) hypothesized origins and maintaining factors for presenting problems, and (4) treatment goals and plans. Additionally, the formulation might include skill deficits and behavioral excesses and deficits, cognitive style or content, typical coping style, among other factors, as well as working models or hypotheses about factors contributing to client difficulties (see Farmer & Chapman, 2008, 2016; Persons & Tompkins, 2007). Based on a clear individual case formulation, the clinician can answer some of the following key questions about phone coaching:

- How will phone coaching enhance therapy outcomes for this client?
- What is my rationale for using phone coaching in view of this client's problem areas and my formulation of the maintaining factors for these problems?
- Is there any reason to think that phone coaching might be contraindicated with this client?
- What role should phone coaching play in this client's treatment?
- How will phone coaching help this client reach her or his goals?
- What is the client's level of skill acquisition, and how will phone coaching enhance generalization for this client?

When to Use Phone Coaching in Standard DBT

It may seem as if phone coaching should always be used in standard DBT, as it's one of the four modes of treatment in DBT. There are times, however, when the clinician may decide not to do phone coaching or to change how it's done with particular clients. In making this decision, one key consideration has to do with the client's stage of treatment.

In DBT, there are four stages. The first stage involves helping the client achieve a reasonable degree of behavioral control and lay the foundation for a good quality of life (often referred to as a "life worth living"; Linehan, 1993a). This often involves eliminating suicidal and self-injurious behaviors and other dysregulated or potentially damaging behavior. The second stage often involves helping the client learn how to effectively experience and accept emotions and thoughts, and may involve work on posttraumatic stress or inhibited grieving (sadness or grief that has, so far, generally been suppressed or avoided). The third stage involves helping the client navigate ordinary problems in his or her life, such as work or relationship stress, difficulties with achieving satisfaction with his or her life, or other normative difficulties. Finally, the fourth stage involves helping the client work on what might be considered more existential issues of meaning and fulfillment. Goals in this stage often are to help the client increase his or her capacity for joy and freedom.

Phone coaching may be used more, less, or differently at different stages of DBT. In stage one, the client in standard DBT receives both individual therapy and group skills training. Phone coaching during this stage is essential and helps the client generalize and integrate the skills she is learning into everyday life. In stage two, the client may no longer be in skills training, and treatment, while based on foundational principles of DBT, may appear a lot more like standard CBT or like mindfulness- or acceptance-oriented approaches. In this stage, the generalization of skills to daily life remains important, but phone coaching may or may not play a major role in this. It is also possible that the client in stage two has now reached the point where it is reasonable to fade out phone coaching in order to encourage the client to develop more sustainable ways to use skills outside sessions. This topic is the focus of Chapter 9. Phone coaching is less likely to be a core component of DBT in stages three and four compared with stages one and two.

The clinician's case formulation and ongoing experiences with the client should also inform her decisions about whether and how to use phone coaching. One clinician was seeing a client transferred from someone else. In his previous therapy, the client struggled to use phone coaching appropriately despite great efforts on the part of the clinician. Although the current therapist was confident that she could manage these issues and help the client learn to use phone coaching effectively, it became apparent that phone coaching may actually have contributed to the worsening of the client's problems. Moreover, the aim of therapy was not to improve the client's phone-coaching behavior, but rather to help him improve the rest of his life. The clinician, therefore, decided not to make phone coaching part of her treatment with this client. Fortunately, the client was nonsuicidal and showed evidence of using skills in his everyday life; thus, instead of phone coaching, the clinician and client emphasized other ways to continue to encourage the generalization of DBT skills.

Another colleague had a client who went through one 6-month cycle of skills training and picked up the skills extremely well. She successfully used interpersonal effectiveness skills in heated and challenging relationship conflicts, had learned to act opposite to her fear of speaking up in meetings at work (something that had led to problems in previous jobs), and had begun to broaden her social network. She was moving steadily toward accomplishing many of her therapy goals, but she still suffered from persistent feelings of loneliness and alienation. As a result, she called the therapist about three or four times per week. Although the therapist was fine with this frequency of calls, he noticed that the majority of phone coaching calls simply helped the client feel a little less lonely for a few minutes. It was clear that the client knew which skills to use and how to use them, even for loneliness, but she had a hard time letting go of phone coaching as a way to feel connected to someone. As a result, the clinician and client decided that the client needed to take a break from phone coaching. Instead, the therapist would periodically call the client in a noncontingent and random manner. Some weeks, he called her twice, and other weeks not at all. The client agreed to use skills and follow their established crisis plan, as she still periodically felt suicidal or had urges to harm herself. In therapy sessions, the dyad worked on building her social supports, encouraging her to contact others in her social network when she felt the need for connection.

In both of these examples, it was most effective to either abandon or modify phone coaching to meet the individual client's needs. Although standard DBT nearly always includes phone coaching, there are cases in which the client (and clinician) may be better off without it. When this is the case, it is important to orient the client to the rationale for any decisions involving the exclusion or modification of phone coaching. I have heard (and used) many creative strategies to make phone coaching work effectively in the context of individual clients' needs and challenges. I will discuss some additional examples later, in Chapter 9, focused on strategies to observe limits and navigate challenges.

Determining How Phone Coaching Fits within Your Practice

Another practical consideration has to do with how phone coaching fits within the structure of your practice setting. In some settings, phone coaching is either not feasible (e.g., in correctional or some other institutional settings) or against agency policy. In my experience training clinicians in DBT, there is sometimes some wiggle room regarding policy when the agency is invested in improved care for complex clients. Although DBT implementation issues are not the focus of this book, particularly effective arguments for DBT programs containing all elements (including phone coaching) involve evidence of the clinical (for a review, see Stoffers et al., 2012) and cost-effectiveness (for a review, see Linehan, Kanter, & Comtois, 1999) of this treatment in reducing suicidal behavior and hospital admissions. Improved efficiency and effectiveness in the care of complex, suicidal clients generally tend to be a goal with which most agencies resonate.

The challenge, then, is to explain how phone coaching fits within an efficient treatment that is clinically and cost-effective. Anecdotally, I have observed that, without phone coaching, many of my clients likely would have gone to the hospital much more frequently. Phone coaching helps clients use skills to avert a crisis or to manage one without resorting to self-injury, suicidal, or other problematic behaviors. If the client needs continued support to avoid engaging in self-destructive behaviors or ending up in the hospital, the clinician can often provide this support. Without phone coaching, clients are left to seek support from crisis lines (often after the crisis hits and suicidality is elevated), other practitioners, or those in their social support network, and suicidal talk in any of these contexts might trigger unnecessary efforts to get the client into the hospital. Hospitalization is expensive and resource-intensive, and there is little evidence for the effectiveness of hospitalization with suicidal patients (Hawton et al., 1999). Therefore, one good argument for the cost-effectiveness of phone coaching is that it may divert clients from the hospital.

In settings where there is flexibility to use phone coaching as indicated with particular clients, clinicians need to make decisions regarding how out-of-session communication fits within the fee structure of the clinic. Ideally, clients will be oriented to these decisions (see sections later in this chapter), and details will be explained in any informed consent documents. At the DBT Centre of Vancouver, for example, we inform clients that they are entitled to 15 minutes of free phone coaching per week, and that they may be billed at their standard individual therapy session rate (prorated for the duration of the phone contact) for phone coaching exceeding 15 minutes in any given week. In reality, many of our clinicians offer much more than 15 minutes free of charge, and I think we've rarely billed clients for phone coaching. We ask clients to agree to this fee arrangement, however, so that we could use it if clinically indicated or desired by the clinician (i.e., payment for extra phone coaching time may increase the clinician's willingness to provide phone coaching). Other clinics neither include a limit nor charge clients for phone coaching, or they charge a higher rate for DBT compared with other services, to account for extra time spent on phone coaching. When it is up to the individual clinician, it is important to decide whether she or he is willing to work outside of regularly scheduled sessions without being paid for the time. A contingency whereby clients are billed for at least a portion of their phone coaching may reduce the likelihood that clients will call too frequently or for reasons that fall outside typical guidelines for skills coaching (e.g., calling to alleviate loneliness or just to chat). It is important to work out all of these issues ahead of time, communicate them clearly to the client, and include them in any relevant fee agreements or informed consent materials.

Considering Personal and Professional Limits Regarding Phone Coaching

Clinicians also should consider how available to their clients they are willing to be between sessions. As mentioned in Chapter 1, in standard DBT, therapists typically are always available to their clients, but the safety valve is that they should always observe their limits and treat as therapy-interfering behavior any occasions when the client is calling too much or making it hard to sustain phone coaching (see Chapter 8; see also Chapman & Rosenthal, 2016; Linehan, 1993a). Although we do not encourage rigid limit setting in DBT, it can be helpful for clinicians to start phone coaching with at least a rough idea of these limits, such as their preferred plan for availability during weekdays and weekends, approximately how many calls they might be willing to fit in, and so forth. Therefore, preparatory consideration of limits should be considered much like drawing a line in pencil on a piece of paper. The line can be erased and changed at any time, but having it there can help the clinician track when a client is crossing it.

As a psychologist with experience with phone coaching, I would like to have done some of this preparatory thinking before I first jumped in. When I first began phone coaching, I was on my predoctoral clinical psychology internship, and I was excited about getting experience with comprehensive DBT. I thought I was ready to dive into phone coaching, and I was looking forward to seeing what it was like to coach clients on skills between sessions. Unfortunately, I had not carefully considered how phone coaching might fit into my everyday life, and I was not prepared for the process of observing my limits. During my first couple of weeks, however, a client started calling me every day of the week and multiple times over the weekend, nearly always when he was experiencing intense, overwhelming emotions or was in a crisis. I took these calls diligently for the first few weeks but noticed that I was feeling increasingly stressed, overwhelmed, and resentful of these calls. I had begun to develop an aversive conditioned response to the specific beeping sound of my pager. It was only a few weeks into my internship, and already I was noticing the signs of burnout! Something had to change, or I would probably start making some crisis calls of my own. When I raised this issue with the client (observing limits, discussed throughout this book but most specifically in Chapter 9), he initially felt frustrated, afraid that he would be without the support he needed, and ashamed that he had been pushing my limits. As it turned out, this pattern of seeking more support than others were willing to provide occurred in other relationships, including previous therapy relationships. Fortunately, we were able to talk through the situation and collaboratively make an arrangement that worked better for both of us. This situation surrounding phone coaching was an important learning experience for both of us. That said, I believe I could have avoided a fair amount of stress if I had given more thought to the process and been more attentive to early signs that the client was asking for more than I was willing to give. Below are some important questions I would like to have asked myself.

"When will I be most willing to take phone coaching calls?"

"What are the early warning signs that phone coaching is going beyond my limits?"

"How many phone coaching calls per week would I likely be willing and able to fit in?"

"What will I do if my client were to call more often than I wish?"

"What will I do if my client were to call repeatedly in a crisis?"

"What arrangements might I need to make to incorporate phone coaching into my professional and personal life?"

As mentioned in Chapter 3, if a clinician has considered these questions and preexisting limits, these should be discussed with the client. That way, the client will have a good idea of when the clinician is most likely and willing to be available. Clinicians treating complex, suicidal clients also should discuss the resources their clients can access or the coping skills they can use when the clinician is unavailable. I have yet to encounter a client who can limit suicidality, crises, or emotional challenges to the hours of 9:00 A.M. to 5:00 P.M. The clinician must use her or his own judgment, expertise, and formulation of the individual case to plan effectively for any necessary between-session care that goes beyond her or his limits.

What about Electronic Communication?

My wife and I were in a restaurant recently, and I saw a father and his preteen daughter enjoying a meal together. Except they weren't enjoying the meal *together*: the father was glued to his smartphone for nearly the whole time, only periodically looking up to respond to something his daughter was saying. I think many of us would agree that electronic communication methods and devices have, for better or worse, infiltrated our lives. This state of affairs raises issues for clinicians practicing phone coaching.

With the capacity for immediate communication with smartphones, expectations are raised that we are all available at all times of day or night. Few among us don't expect an immediate response to a text. The same expectations hold true for clients, raising their expectations that they will receive a response to a text within moments. They assume you've seen a message and will respond quickly. They may feel upset, frustrated, confused, or hurt if they don't hear from you. It is important to consider how you might handle these types of situations. Moreover, many clients e-mail about their problems or what happened in a previous session and can expect clinicians to read and respond quickly to their e-mails.

Clinicians deciding ahead of time on their limits around electronic communication can avoid potential conflict and therapy-interfering behavior. Although the clinician's limits may change throughout treatment, starting with clearly defined limits with clients can help to prevent problems. In my experience, therapy burnout related to electronic communication often results primarily from failure to specify, orient the client to, and observe limits. Bob, for example, had generally used e-mail and text messaging judiciously with his clients, and his clients usually e-mailed and texted appropriately and not too frequently. There really wasn't any reason in Bob's mind for concern about e-mailing and texting with his clients. When he started working with Sally, his attitude had to change. Sally started off by simply calling him occasionally, but after a month or so, she began texting and e-mailing multiple times per day, regularly asking for urgent assistance over text (e.g., texting in the middle of a crisis or emergency, when suicidal, and so on), and e-mailing lengthy messages about the therapy relationship or reactions to what Bob had said in session. Bob felt demoralized by this onslaught of electronic communication and began to notice the signs of burnout. By this point, Sally had become so used to frequent communication with Bob that it was very difficult for her to change her behavior. Moreover, when Bob raised the issue, Sally became angry and refused to discuss it. Bob began to feel as if wasps were swarming around him. He was overwhelmed with the sheer quantity and different forms of Sally's communication, and whenever he tried to make changes to the situation (i.e., wave the wasps away), he got stung. While this may be an extreme case, many clinicians who don't prepare ahead of time can quickly become overwhelmed with electronic communication. This is why it is so important to consider several questions before embarking upon phone coaching via text or e-mail.

- "Am I willing to e-mail or text regarding personal or clinical information with clients?"
- "What are my limits in terms of how often or when I am willing to receive or respond to e-mails or texts?"
- "How promptly am I willing to read and respond to e-mails or texts?"

- "What are my limits in terms of the content of text messages or e-mails from clients (e.g., texts or e-mails regarding suicidality, extensive information about clinical issues)?"
- "What are the ethical issues, such as confidentiality, that I need to consider regarding electronic communication?"
- "If a client is e-mailing, what server or system stores her e-mails and my e-mails, and what are the potential threats to the security of confidential information?"
- "Do I need to include copies of electronic communication in the client's clinical file?"

Potential Advantages and Disadvantages of Electronic Communication

There are several potential advantages of the use of electronic communication for skills coaching. Texting requires little effort. When a longer phone conversation is not possible, the clinician can be available via text to respond quickly to brief questions or to provide suggestions or encouragement. Text messaging also is useful to remind clients to practice certain skills; provide brief, supportive messages; and so on. E-mail can provide the client with the opportunity to thoughtfully describe his experiences in a way that might be difficult to do on the spot during a phone call or an individual therapy session. I have had some clients who were initially reluctant to engage in phone coaching due to anxiety and shame. Using shaping principles, it was helpful to begin with e-mail coaching and proceed to a greater emphasis on phone coaching. Furthermore, electronic communication broadens the range and media through which clients and clinicians can communicate. Clients are able to communicate and express themselves through photos, drawings, music, quotes, brief statements (like "tweets"), and so on. This is consistent with how many people communicate these days. Furthermore, clients can easily save and later access electronic communication with the clinician to remind themselves of useful tips and ideas. Thus, electronic communication may facilitate the generalization of skills and knowledge to the client's everyday life. As I discuss in a later chapter, I regularly e-mail reminders to group-skills-training clients about homework, and provide them with inspiring quotes that are relevant to the skills they're learning, helpful suggestions, and so forth. Several clients have remarked that they find these messages helpful and often save and revisit certain passages or quotes.

Despite these advantages, electronic communication can create numerous problems. Because it is so easy to quickly text, clients may learn to seek support from their therapist without bothering to try the skills they're learning. Some clients are more likely to seek the immediate gratification of a supportive text message from their therapist than to open up their skills binders, look through and consider which skills to use, and try them out before contacting the clinician.

Many people also have grown accustomed to using text, e-mail, or other messaging forums in a fairly unstructured, unmindful, and non-goal-oriented manner. This is perfectly understandable and normative; however, phone coaching has clear goals and ideally is structured to achieve those goals. Many of us have encountered clients who text in a manner that does not fit the principles or goals of phone coaching. Seemingly random texts arrive with unclear statements or requests or include disclosures that sometimes raise ethical or other issues (statements regarding suicide, drug use, urges to quit therapy, etc.), and so forth. It is not always clear how to manage or respond to such communications. Indeed, simply responding may reinforce behavior that is inconsistent with effective phone coaching.

It is also easy for both clinicians and clients to misinterpret the tone or intent of a written message. Many of us have said something over text or e-mail (even to a client) that we would never say in person, or that could be taken the wrong way in the absence of cues such as facial expression or voice tone. Complex clients with relationship challenges may be particularly sensitive to these issues, and the resulting relationship ruptures can take therapy astray. Clinicians are not immune to these reactions. Clients sometimes write things (e.g., overly harsh criticism written in a state of anger) to their clinicians that are harmful to the therapy relationship. I have sometimes been taken off guard with the content or tone of a client's e-mail, feeling frustrated, confused, or hurt in response to something the client likely would never have said in person.

A few additional issues are more specific to e-mail. One potential concern is that clients may use e-mail as a substitute for in-person or telephone communication. I find it much easier to be helpful when I have a chance to interact in person or on the phone with clients (granted, this could be because I did not grow up as part of an electronics-focused generation); thus, I do not prefer e-mail or text messaging as a substitute for phone communication. If I were temporarily using e-mail with a client reluctant to call, and she was unable to progress to coaching over the phone, I would address this issue as a potentially therapy-interfering behavior and collaboratively determine how to help the client use the phone for skills coaching.

E-mail also allows clients to write a lot more than they would normally say. This is not always a good thing. Many of us have worked with clients who send extremely lengthy e-mails between sessions and expect the clinician to have read these thoroughly every week. Given how busy I am and the huge volume of e-mails I receive daily, this goes beyond my limits, but other clinicians may be comfortable with this arrangement. Clinicians considering phone coaching or other forms of between-session communication should consider their limits regarding these issues and communicate them clearly to the client. In Chapter 3 I discuss orientation to clinician limits, and in Chapter 8 I discuss ways to observe them.

The Confidentiality and Ethics of Electronic Communication

Also important to consider is the confidentiality of electronic communication. It is difficult to ensure the privacy or confidentiality of electronic communication. In some ways, this may be a greater concern for the clinician than for the client, given that the sharing of personal information broadly over social networking has become normative. Nevertheless, as mental health professionals, we are obligated to let clients know what they're getting into when they communicate with us electronically. I recommend that the reader consider guidelines from the American Psychological Association (APA, 1997; Lannin & Scott, 2014), the Canadian Psychological Association (CPA; 2006), and/or other local associations regarding electronic communication. Drude and Lichstein (2005) also have published a very helpful article on issues in the use of e-mail with clients. It is also important to review regulations put forth by local licensing boards regarding electronic communication, confidentiality, and documentation issues. Where I practice, for example, we must save all electronic communication (including texts) in the client's file. Some clinicians might opt out of electronic communication simply because of the time commitment associated with this administrative work. I'm not interested in spending moments of my life copying, PDF'ing, printing, or uploading texts or e-mails to client files, and I sometimes provide this sense of wasting time as part of my rationale for avoiding electronic communication for clinical issues.

Ensuring Adequate Support and Consultation

I will assume for the purposes of this section that the clinician is an independently licensed or registered practitioner. Students and trainees practicing phone coaching under supervision hopefully already have in place adequate regular supervision and/or consultation. For those clinicians who are seeing many complex, multiproblem clients or who regularly take suicide crisis calls, a supportive team or system of consultation is essential. Both during phone coaching and within therapy more broadly, it can be easy to go astray with complex and challenging clients. The pressure and stress associated with work with suicidal individuals can, at times, be overwhelming. Clinicians may also deviate from effective phone coaching practices out of caring for the client or because it is difficult to manage contingencies or maintain reasonable limits. It can be easy to get stuck in the forest so to speak and not be able to see the landmarks suggesting that phone coaching is going down the wrong path.

The DBT Consultation Team Model

In DBT, the primary way to provide clinicians with support and maintain motivation and skill is the *DBT consultation team* (Linehan, 1993a). The consultation team, one of the four primary modes of standard DBT (including individual therapy, phone coaching, skills training, and consultation team), involves a weekly meeting focused on clinician behaviors, emotions, thoughts, skills, and motivation in relation to their work with complex clients. In contrast with a traditional supervision or case conference meeting, the consultation team meeting is much more like "therapy for the clinicians." To facilitate open disclosure and help seeking on the part of clinicians, all members of consult teams are treated as peers. Although the particular context for a consult team may include built-in hierarchies (employers, supervisors, registrants, nonregistrants, trainees, etc.), meetings are conducted in such a manner as to reduce the influence of these hierarchies. Each clinician must feel free to disclose challenges in her or his work with minimal fear of judgment or negative consequences to her or his status or position. Naturally, any applicable ethical and professional standards, laws, and codes of conduct may, at times, limit any consultation team's ability to fully actualize this peer-focused philosophy.

Having a DBT consultation team in place can help clinicians to navigate phone coaching effectively. During DBT consultation team meetings, for example, clinicians are encouraged to put their issues on the agenda if they need help due to a client's therapy-interfering behavior. Therapy-interfering behaviors during phone coaching (discussed more extensively in Chapter 8) may include the client calling too much, acting in a defensive or hostile manner on the phone, being unwilling to accept coaching suggestions or to talk about skills, using phone coaching for purposes other than coaching, staying too long on the phone, using electronic communication in a manner that goes beyond the clinician's limits, and so on. Clinicians themselves can also engage in therapy-interfering phone-coaching behaviors, such as allowing phone calls to go on too long or to occur too frequently, failing to appropriately structure the calls, regularly addressing topics other than skills coaching on the phone, failing to get back to the client, responding to unwanted texts or e-mails, and becoming burned out without having taken precautionary measures, among others. The team supports clinicians and helps them find effective solutions if or when these and other difficulties with phone coaching arise. Having a team or a go-to colleague can also be helpful when the clinician needs on-the-spot consultation regarding a client at risk of imminent harm to self or others. Consistent with the dialectical philosophy of DBT, the consultation team helps the clinician figure out whether anything is being left out of her or his conceptualization or care of the client.

In the example provided of Bob and his client Sally, Bob had started to notice that he was feeling burned out, and he put his issue on the agenda of the DBT consultation team. Initially, it wasn't clear to him as to how he had gotten so far down the path to burnout in such a short time, but his team helped him assess the situation and realize that he was stretching his limits. They also helped him come up with solutions and practice effective ways to discuss his problem with Sally. Other examples include clinicians who are so stressed out by a client who is calling frequently that she or he fails to adequately assess, empathize with, or understand the function of the client's repeated calls. The team can help to understand the function of this behavior to help the client change it. A detailed discussion of the DBT consultation team is beyond the scope of this book, but I can say that I have been much more willing to do phone coaching with clients when I've had a DBT consultation team at my disposal. Even if that is not possible, I would highly recommend that clinicians treating complex clients and practicing phone coaching have a supportive system of peer consultation or supervision in place.

Becoming Familiar with Key DBT Principles and Practices Pertaining to Phone Coaching

Another preparation task involves becoming familiar with the DBT principles and practices associated with phone coaching. It is beyond the scope of this book to delve into depth regarding the theoretical underpinnings of DBT or core DBT intervention strategies at great length. While I believe that many readers will be able to begin to implement phone coaching in a manner that is consistent with DBT after carefully reading this book, I would strongly recommend the review of Marsha Linehan's primary DBT manual (Linehan, 1993a), as well as the most recent version of the DBT skills training manual (Linehan, 2015). Other excellent texts on DBT focus on ways to incorporate this treatment into clinical practice (Koerner, 2012), guidelines and principles for the management of suicidal behavior among adolescents (Rathus & Miller, 2014), and several others.

Being Dialectical about Preparing for Phone Coaching

Although I am recommending that the clinician considering phone coaching engage in some significant preparation, there is a key dialectic here to consider. As with any significant therapeutic modality, phone coaching requires preparation to be effective, and clinicians often have little idea of what they need to prepare for until they actually do it. This is true of many activities. If you were to go on a ski trip, you'd certainly make some preparations: make travel arrangements; bring appropriate clothing, ski gear, and money for food; and so forth. Once you're on the mountain, however, shifting weather and snow conditions on the slopes and the presence of crowds and long lift lines will likely teach you what you would like to have prepared for. Each client brings something different to phone coaching. Some clients become attached very quickly and call a lot, whereas others don't call at all. Some clients are extremely appreciative of suggestions regarding skills, and others get angry when their therapists suggest skills. Some therapists start phone coaching with great enthusiasm only to discover later that it's not for them, or that coaching on the fly is not their strong suit. Therefore, like many tasks in life, preparation is essential, and reality is often quite different from the situation we might have prepared so much for.

Summary

Laying the groundwork for effective phone coaching involves preparation at both motivational and logistical levels. The clinician should begin by considering her or his commitment to use phone coaching. Clinicians should also consider for whom phone coaching would be beneficial. Other preparatory tasks are practical, such as determining how phone coaching will fit within the clinician's practice. If the clinician is working in a private practice setting, how does phone coaching fit in terms of the clinician's fee structure? If the clinician is working for an agency, how will the clinician navigate phone coaching in that context? Clinicians also need to decide about how to make decisions regarding any preferred parameters and limits around phone coaching and how electronic communication methods might be used. Clinicians seeing complex clients and conducting phone coaching ideally should have in place a supportive consultation network or team. Finally, effective DBT phone coaching requires the clinician to be familiar with the principles, theory, and practices of DBT pertaining to phone coaching as well as with the DBT skills (Linehan, 1993b, 2015). A clinician considering the use of this potentially useful intervention mode should consider these practical issues and plan carefully.

CHAPTER 3

Orientation to Phone Coaching

O nce a clinician has decided to use phone coaching, the next step is to provide the client with a thorough *orientation* to this mode of treatment. Orientation involves explaining to the client the rationale, procedures, and rules associated with phone coaching. When conducted effectively, orientation to any therapeutic procedure or intervention provides the client with clear expectations regarding the roles and expected behavior of the client and the clinician. When the client is aware of why phone coaching is important, what to do when she or he calls the clinician, and what to expect of the clinician, phone coaching often proceeds smoothly and effectively. Indeed, clear and thorough orientation prevents many common problems from arising in therapy. The focus of this chapter is on ways to effectively orient clients to phone coaching.

Provide a Rationale

Providing a rationale that emphasizes coaching as a way to generalize skills can help the client understand when and why to call. The primary purpose of phone coaching is to *generalize* skills the client is learning in therapy to her or his natural environment. Coaching in real-world, ongoing, challenging situations is the primary way in which the clinician using phone coaching helps the client generalize new learning. It is important, therefore, for clients to know that phone coaching will focus on the use of skills in their natural, everyday environments.

Clients may call their clinicians for a variety of reasons, including loneliness, the desire to connect to someone, a perceived need for reassurance, to solve major problems in life (such as a dysfunctional relationship), to get help in a crisis or emergency, and so forth. Some of these reasons to call are consistent with the goals of coaching and generalization, and others are not. Calls stemming from loneliness, for example, would not be consistent with the goals of coaching and generalization if contact with the clinician is the client's primary method of alleviating loneliness. To bring a loneliness-related call in line with generalization and coaching, the clinician would need to actively coach the client on how to find ways to alleviate or tolerate loneliness in the short term (i.e., during next few hours to next few days). In the longer term, the dyad may work on loneliness in their individual therapy sessions. Arguably, calling a clinician to alleviate loneliness involves the skill of reaching out for support. The clinician and client, therefore, could work on ways to generalize that skill beyond the therapy relationship. The primary focus of phone coaching calls, therefore, should be on active coaching on the use of generalizable skills. Understanding this principle and rationale helps clients to comprehend that calls are not simply meant for talking. Rather, they can expect their clinician to actively focus on coaching and skills. If the client is not seeking skills coaching, it may be effective to meet her or his needs through means other than a telephone call (or text, e-mail, and so on) with the clinician.

Below is a dialogue in which a clinician orients a client to the rationale and purpose of phone coaching:

THERAPIST: Now that we've agreed to work together, I'd like to spend some time discussing an important part of our work.

CLIENT: OK, what is that?

THERAPIST: Well, as you might have noticed, the problems that bring you to therapy are not simple or easily solved. Would you agree?

CLIENT: True, I mean I've been struggling for so long, and it's not like I haven't tried other therapy before.

THERAPIST: Exactly, and given how bright and capable you are, I'm pretty sure you would have solved your problems already if they weren't so complex. Well, when you have complex problems, you need a comprehensive kind of therapy. This means a therapy where you get help in many areas. Remember how we've talked about skills training as an important part of therapy?

CLIENT: Yeah, that's the group, right?

THERAPIST: Yes, you'll be starting the skills training group on Tuesday, and I think you're going to find it extremely helpful. That group is all about learning new skills—strategies you can use to manage your emotions, live effectively in the present moment, deal with other people, and ride out crises. In fact, this whole therapy is all about learning new things. One way to help you bring these new skills into your life is for me to be there to assist you when you really need help—like when you are not sure what skill to use or how to use it. Does that make sense?

CLIENT: Sure, but how are you going to do that? Are you planning on stalking me?

THERAPIST: Ha! No, definitely not, but I am planning on giving you my cell phone number so that you can call me when you need help. In DBT, we call this "phone coaching." You can call me when you're in need of coaching on when, how, or why to use skills to cope with difficult situations.

CLIENT: Oh, that sounds really helpful. My other clinician only took calls about scheduling appointments. I normally had to call the crisis line for help in an emergency.

THERAPIST: In our work, the idea would be to call me if you need help using skills in everyday life. I believe that doing this regularly will help you to bring the therapy into your life. That's the main purpose of the calls. They're not meant to be crisis calls. In fact, I'd encourage you to call me well before a crisis hits. That way, we can find a way for you to use skills to prevent the crisis.

CLIENT: That sounds like a good idea. So, I can't call you in an emergency?

THERAPIST: You can, and that is one of the three reasons to call me that we'll talk about in a few minutes. But, as I've said, it would be better to call me before an emergency rather than in the middle of one. That's because you're better off learning how to avoid getting into emergencies or crisis than just learning how to manage them. We do also have skills, though, to help you manage crises, and we'll go through those as well.

Clarify That Phone Coaching Is Not Therapy or a Crisis Service

Given that phone coaching may be a new modality to clients, it is important to explain the difference between phone coaching and therapy. This clarification can help the client understand how to approach phone coaching calls. I often tell clients that phone coaching is a lot like coaching on the fly in hockey or other sports. The coach is there to provide quick feedback, suggestions, and directives to improve the gameplay in the moment, but there is no time to discuss strategy, analyze performance, or plan to dig the team out of a losing streak. I let the client know that I'm going to focus mainly on how to use skills to regulate or tolerate emotions occurring in the context of a challenging situation. We probably won't be able to solve the problem or work on the long-term goals that brought the client to therapy. As mentioned in Chapter 1, coaching guides the client in effective directions when she or he is unsure of which skills to use or how to use them. I tell clients that calls will usually be 5–10 minutes in length, and that it will be important to get down to business fairly quickly. There is usually no time to process interactions between the client and the clinician, work on longer-term life goals, talk about aspects of one's past history, or to simply vent or express feelings or opinions at length. Because some clients are very sensitive to changes in their therapist's demeanor or style, I sometimes let clients know ahead of time that I might be more task-oriented on the phone than I am in our regular sessions.

It is also helpful to convey to the client that phone coaching is not a suicide or self-injury prevention or crisis call service; it is a skills coaching service. Orienting the client to this point will help to cut down on the number of calls related to crises or emergencies and will hopefully result in the client calling in advance for help in averting such situations. One early mistake (one of many) I made in phone coaching was telling a client to call me when he felt like self-injuring or engaging in suicidal behavior. This is an easy mistake for beginning DBT clinicians to make. Or, at least, that's what I've told myself. Telling a client to call when she or he is feeling self-injurious or suicidal can result in an excessive number of calls, or establish a contingency whereby the client receives more help and support when she or he is suicidal or self-injurious than at other times. In the worst-case scenario, the client learns (with or without awareness) to become suicidal or self-injurious in order to receive support or attention.

In my case, the client began to call me whenever he had significant urges to self-injure, which was nearly daily. He usually felt better after our calls, used distress tolerance skills, and avoided cutting himself. In some ways, however, our calls had become his substitute for self-injury, as he found them reassuring and soothing. I had to take a step back and tell this client that the deal was not for him to call me whenever he had significant urges to self-injure. I told him I was confident that he could get through those urges most of the time. I wanted to hear from him, however, when he was in a difficult situation (or possibly anticipating one) and not sure what skills to use or how to use them. Uncoupling the calls from self-injury urges took time, but after about a month, the client was consistently using other skills to manage these urges, and the frequency of calls had reduced to about one or two every couple of weeks.

Explaining When and Why to Call

The clinician should also provide the client with clear guidelines on when to call. As briefly mentioned in Chapter 1, in DBT there are three primary reasons for phone coaching calls. The first and primary reason to call is for *skills coaching*—assistance in determining when and how to use certain skills. As discussed and illustrated above, skills coaching is the primary purpose of phone coaching, and this fact should be made clear to the client. In the therapy example above, the clinician makes the distinction between calls focused on skills coaching and calls focused on emergencies or crises.

Notwithstanding, another reason for clients to call the clinician is for *help in an emergency or crisis*. Writings on standards of care for suicidal patients emphasize the importance of between-session support (Bongar, Sheykhani, Kugel, & Giannini, 2015). It is hard to imagine how complex, suicidal clients will receive maximal benefit from treatment that only occurs in the therapy office, or that doesn't include real-time help navigating crises or overwhelming situations. Help during a crisis from a trained clinician who is familiar with one's life circumstances, key problem areas, skills and skill deficits, and treatment plan is likely to be more effective than assistance from a crisis line volunteer (although this is indeed a hypothesis that should be tested). When I orient clients to this reason for phone coaching, however, I clarify that (1) a long-term goal is to minimize crises, (2) calls well in advance of a crisis are likely to be most helpful, and (3) repeated crisis calls will likely interfere with therapy; thus, we will try to reduce them.

A third standard reason for phone coaching in DBT is to discuss *issues in the therapy relationship*. Clinicians orient clients so that they may call the clinician if a difficult therapy relationship issue might simmer over the course of the week or make it hard for the client to attend or tolerate the next session. In orienting about this reason for phone coaching, it is helpful for the clinician to provide examples of relationship issues that might give rise to a phone coaching call. Below are some common examples:

- Strong emotional reactions to something the clinician has said, or the manner in which the clinician said it, such as her voice tone or demeanour.
- Behavior on the part of the clinician that the client finds distressing or disrespectful, such as the clinician arriving late and failing to apologize or being inattentive, critical, or invalidating.
- Ruptures in the therapy relationship, which could include a variety of situations, some examples of which are that the clinician and client are not on the same page regarding goals, the clinician has been pushing the client to change and the client feels misunderstood, and so forth.

It is essential to clarify that these relationship-oriented calls, as with other phone coaching calls, will focus on skills to manage or tolerate difficult emotions. Phone coaching is unlikely to solve challenging relationship problems. Extended discussions, heart-to-heart talks, or problem solving can occur as needed in the next therapy session. In the meantime, the relationship-oriented call is a stopgap measure to help the client cope effectively until the problem can be addressed more thoroughly.

Sometimes, clients will call and say they would like to quit therapy. I consider quitting therapy to be a solution to some kind of problem in therapy. The problem might be that therapy is not working as the client would like it to; the client is upset with me; logistical issues (e.g., work schedule, finances) are hampering the client's therapy attendance; and so forth. I prefer to take time in a therapy session to assess and understand the problem or problems contributing to urges to quit and to collaboratively consider a range of solutions. Clearly, phone coaching is not the forum for discussion of whether to quit therapy. Therefore, if my client calls to discuss the desire to quit, has regularly reported urges to quit therapy, or has a history of quitting other therapies, I will orient her to defer to our next therapy session any discussions of whether to quit therapy. If the client does call to discuss this issue, I will often say something like, "You're not allowed to quit on the phone, and this is a big topic that we'll have to discuss next time we meet. In the meantime, how can I help you with skills coaching?" Sometimes, in these circumstances, skills coaching focuses on how to help the client tolerate distress associated with waiting until the next therapy session to discuss the problems prompting her urges to quit.

Below is an example of a clinician making some of the points discussed in this section while orienting a client to the main reasons to call.

THERAPIST: So, generally, there are three main reasons to call me. The most common reason is that you need help with skills coaching. This means you're dealing with a challenging situation, and you're not sure what skills to use or how to use them. Does that make sense?

CLIENT: Yeah, kind of like when I saw that Facebook post of my boyfriend with another woman at that restaurant, and I kind of lost it.

THERAPIST: That would be a good example. If we had a chance to chat, we could have talked about skills for you to deal with the emotions that came up in that situation. That's the focus of phone coaching— skills to tolerate or regulate emotions. We can't solve big life problems with phone coaching, but we can help you tolerate or manage your emotions until we get a chance to work on those problems together. So, that's the first reason: Call when you want phone coaching. The second reason to call is if something has come up between us that you're having a hard time with.

CLIENT: I'm not sure what you mean by that.

THERAPIST: Well, let's say I said something in one of our sessions, and you felt hurt, confused, criticized, or the like. Or, you have some concerns about how we're working together that would be hard to put off until our next session. In these cases, we can have a quick call to discuss skills to cope with stuff happening in our therapy. Have you ever had something come up—whether it's something someone said, or just their voice tone or something—where you ended up stewing or ruminating about it for a while afterward?

CLIENT: Absolutely, that's probably the main reason I'm here. I'm really sensitive to how people say things and what they say. I wish I wasn't, and I know it doesn't make any sense, but . . .

THERAPIST: I can see what you mean. It can be painful and frustrating to be really sensitive. And what happens if you just keep stewing and avoid talking to the person?

CLIENT: Things usually blow up, like I get really mad the next time I see the person, or I just stay away and avoid the person.

THERAPIST: Many of us have fallen into that trap from time to time. We don't want that happening with us. That's exactly why it's important to call. Now, you don't need to call every time you feel a strong reaction to something in one of our sessions. Just call if you need skills to avoid allowing it to stew and build up over the week. Are you willing to do that?

CLIENT: Yeah, that sounds good. If I had to call someone every time I felt hurt, I'd be on the phone all day!

THERAPIST: Good point! OK, so the third reason to call is if you are in an emergency or crisis. This might mean that you feel totally overwhelmed and in a horribly stressful situation. It might also mean that you're suicidal or likely to hurt yourself or someone else. Now, I just want to be clear: We don't want to have very many of these types of calls.

CLIENT: Why?

THERAPIST: Because I'm a lot more helpful before the crisis hits and well before you become really suicidal. Once you're really suicidal, I can help you lower your risk and avoid making things worse for yourself, but I'd rather help you prevent a crisis and use skills before you get too far down the path to a crisis.

CLIENT: OK, that makes sense.

THERAPIST: So, that means that if we regularly have crisis calls, we're going to talk about how to make things go differently—how you can catch problems before they become so big and call me for help then. Are you willing to agree to that?

CLIENT: I can do my best. I can't promise that I won't call you in a crisis. Sometimes, they just happen so quickly.

THERAPIST: Of course, I get that. I expect my clients to sometimes call in a crisis. It's important, though, to learn how to avoid getting onto the path to a crisis. Does that sound reasonable?

CLIENT: Yes, I think I get it.

Orient Clients to the 24-Hour Rule

Orienting clients to the *24-hour rule* is essential but sometimes challenging. Some clients understand and agree with this rule, whereas others have negative reactions. I've had clients who thought the 24-hour rule was presumptuous, patronizing, or based on a misconception that the client self-injures or attempts suicide simply to cry for help. Other clients have expressed the concern that this rule prevents them from getting help to reduce ongoing risk following an episode of self-injury or a suicide attempt. Although clear orientation often assuages these concerns, some clients remained concerned. If so, I recommend that the clinician validate any reasonable concerns as well as the fact that it's frustrating to have a rule you disagree with imposed on you, but ultimately proceed with the 24-hour rule in place anyway. Below is an example of a clinician orienting a client to the 24-hour rule:

THERAPIST: Phone coaching has an important rule that we should discuss.

CLIENT: Oh, OK.

THERAPIST: This is called the 24-hour rule. The rule is that we can't communicate by phone (or e-mail, text, or whatever) for 24 hours after you self-injure or attempt suicide. So, if you've harmed yourself, I won't be available for phone coaching for at least 24 hours. This rule does not apply to therapy sessions. So, even if you harm yourself on Tuesday evening, you can't get out of seeing me on Wednesday morning!

CLIENT: This sounds kind of harsh. Why do you have that rule?

THERAPIST: Well, the main reason is that I want to avoid unintentionally increasing your risk of self-injury or suicide. If you talk with me right after harming yourself, your brain might make a connection between self-injury and help or support from me. Can you see how this might increase your risk?

CLIENT: I guess. Is it like I'm getting a reward or attention or something?

THERAPIST: You've got it. If you self-harm or try to kill yourself and something good happens, you might be more likely to do it again. This is what we call "positive reinforcement." Self-injury and suicide are like any other behavior. If you get some kind of bonus from doing them, you're more likely to do them again. I know you've said that you sometimes feel better after hurting yourself. So, the bonus you normally get is that you get away from certain emotions. Correct?

CLIENT: Yeah, I'd say that's my main reason to cut. I mean, usually the anger and other stuff, like feeling really agitated, goes away.

THERAPIST: That's the most common reason people say they hurt themselves or attempt suicide. It's also another type of reinforcement: negative reinforcement. Something you don't want goes away when you hurt yourself. Because of that, you're more likely to keep hurting yourself. The reason for the 24-hour rule is that I don't want to reinforce your self-injury or suicide attempts. Does that make sense?

CLIENT: That's not why I hurt myself, though. As I said, I usually do it to feel better. I'm not some kind of drama queen! I don't cut myself to get attention. I used to hate it when my parents said I did that.

THERAPIST: I can see why you wouldn't like that, and I'm not saying you're doing it on purpose to get attention. But, it's still possible that your brain might make that connection, even without your awareness. Your brain might be like, "I just cut myself, and someone who cares about me is helping me." Your brain is more likely to make that connection if I help you right away, compared to a day or two later. That's something else that we know about behavior, but we'll talk about that later. For now, I just want to be extra careful to avoid even the remote possibility that I might increase your risk. So, the 24-hour rule is about me being extra careful about your safety and well-being. And, I think you probably need that. What do you think?

CLIENT: OK, I can see what you're saying. I don't agree that it would increase my risk, but I see how this is you being careful.

THERAPIST: OK, so let me tell you how this works . . .

In this example, the clinician provides a rationale for the 24-hour rule and discusses the client's concerns and questions. The clinician validates the client's point that her self-injury may have nothing to do with social reinforcement. At the same time, the clinician conveys concern about the possibility, however remote, of his reinforcing her self-injury. As shown in the example, it can be effective to frame the 24-hour rule as a way to be extra cautious and careful. It is difficult (but not impossible!) to argue with someone who says he wants to be especially careful about your safety. In contrast, I have found that the rationale that this is just part of the treatment protocol does not resonate as well with clients. Although DBT and other forms of CBT do indeed have manuals and protocols, when clinicians focus primarily on procedural rationales clients may get the impression that the clinician cares more about the manual than their well-being or is lumping them in with all of the other clients and not treating them as individuals.

THERAPIST: The deal is that you will call me only if you haven't harmed yourself for at least 24 hours.

CLIENT: What if I make a mistake and call you anyway?

THERAPIST: Good question. If you call me, I'll start by reminding you of the 24-hour rule. My priority then will be to check on your safety and whether you might need medical attention. After that, we will end our call.

CLIENT: That sounds a little rough. It would be hard if you hung up on me just because I hurt myself. I mean, this is one of the things I'm here for help with. It's like you're rejecting me for my problems.

THERAPIST: I know it might seem kind of harsh, and it might be hard for both of us if I have to get off the phone with you. In all of my time doing this work, it has only happened a handful of times. Some of those times, I think I had a harder time ending the call than my client did! In any case, it's not like I'll get mad at you or hang up on you right away. But I will politely end the call quite soon. Basically, it won't be a normal phone coaching call.

CLIENT: OK, that makes sense. I just hope it doesn't happen.

THERAPIST: Me too. Think of it this way. You've told me how frustrated you are with the mental health system. It's like you have to be really bad off, delusional, or suicidal to get immediate help, right? That's sort of how you ended up in this program. You get more help if you're suicidal, and you're all alone if you're not. Do you think there might be something wrong with that?

CLIENT: Yeah, it's like things have to get really really bad for me to get help. When things are bad and I'm still miserable but not trying to kill myself, I can't get help.

THERAPIST: So, we're trying to reverse that whole system here. It's the opposite: You get more help when you haven't hurt yourself. I think this is a better way to help you improve your life and solve the problems making you miserable.

Clarify the Expected Length of Calls

As mentioned in Chapter 1, phone coaching calls in DBT are brief, although there is no standard yardstick for the length of these calls. My preference is usually around 5–15 minutes, but this is arbitrary, and sometimes calls go longer (or shorter) by necessity. It is important, however, to make it clear to the client during orientation that calls will be brief. When the client expects the phone call to be brief, he won't be surprised when the clinician needs to end the call or says that certain topics (e.g., issues that take a fair amount of time to work out) are best deferred to a therapy session. I find it helpful to let clients know that we'll do our best to come up with a solid plan, but that our time might run out before we're able to do so. When that is the case, I encourage the client to try to make the best possible use of the coaching we managed to fit in during the call. Beyond orienting clients to the length of calls before first using phone coaching, it is helpful to remind clients of how much time is available at the beginning of each call. I often say something like, "Just so you know, I only have about 10 [or 7, or 5, etc., as the case may be] minutes to talk." In addition, I find it helpful to make some mention of the time remaining about halfway through the call.

Clarify Any Clinician Limits around Phone Coaching

During orientation, the clinician should clarify any important preexisting phone coaching limits or preferences, but I recommend that the clinician be careful not to overemphasize limit setting or institute many rules and specifications for phone coaching. Several times I have seen clinicians attempt to devise rules, contracts, and procedures (often anti-DBT) around phone coaching. This ends up complicating matters, and the clinician has to keep track of the rules (which sometimes differ across clients) and have some way to respond when they're violated. This type of system is not typical of what any of us usually experience in everyday life relationships (e.g., "OK, son, I'll take calls from you but only for 5 minutes and between 2:00 and 5:00 P.M. If you call more often than that, we'll have to revisit this arrangement."). Recall from Chapter 1 that DBT principles emphasize *observing* rather than setting limits. Nevertheless, it is important for clients to know how available the clinician is willing to be, and if there are preexisting limits, these should be clearly outlined. Doing so can prevent confusion and increase the chances that phone coaching will work well for both parties. Below is a brief example of how a clinician might clarify and orient a client to limits around phone coaching (not including electronic communication, which is discussed in the next section).

> "I'll be available by phone for skills coaching most days of the week, unless I tell you otherwise. On some weekdays or weekends, I might have family or work obligations that make my schedule a little more unpredictable, so I might get back to you quickly or slowly on those days. I'll try to let you know ahead of time if I'm unavailable, and if so, I'll have one of my colleagues provide back-up phone coverage. Also, I should let you know that I frequently travel, and I'll usually identify a backup person that you can call when I'm away. This person will be part of our clinical team and will have access to your information so she or he can provide the best possible help to you in my absence. In terms of timing, I'm up fairly early in the morning, usually 5:30 or 6:00 A.M., and I go to bed around 10:00 P.M. If you call outside these hours, it's possible that my phone might not wake me up, or it might not be nearby, and if you catch me in the middle of the night, there's a good chance I won't be as helpful as I usually am. Because of this, we should plan for those times when it might be hard to reach me. Also, you should know that I almost never answer my phone when it rings, so you'll have to leave a very brief voice message describing the kind of help that you need. Because it's so easy for people to accidentally call, and I like to know what kind of help you need before I call you back, I'll only return calls if you leave a voice message. Although I'll try to get back to you as soon as I can, on some days I might call you back within half an hour, and on other days, you might have to wait several hours. I will do my

best to at least get back to you the same day, before I go to bed that night. This means that if you struggle with urges to harm yourself, you will have to agree not to hurt yourself while you wait for my call. During that time, I recommend that you make use of skills from your binder. I know this might be hard, so we'll discuss what to do under these circumstances. I don't have any set number of calls I can take per week, and if you're calling too much or too little, I'll let you know, and we'll work together to make phone coaching work best for both of us. Let's talk about any questions you might have about these arrangements."

Discussing Electronic Communication Methods

Although I don't know that all of my DBT colleagues would agree with me, one area where I believe it's important to clearly define clinician limits ahead of time rather than waiting to observe limits when they're pushed is electronic communication. Stan worked full time as a therapist and had only a few minutes here and there throughout the day to check his e-mail. By the end of the workday, he enjoyed setting the smartphone and computer aside and spending time with loved ones, engaging in recreational activities, and so forth. Although he strongly preferred not to communicate with his clients over text or e-mail (and didn't have much time for it), he did not convey this therapeutic limit at the beginning of his work with Joanie. Joanie, in contrast, was wedded to her smartphone and texted and (to a lesser extent) e-mailed periodically throughout the day. Used to hearing back from people immediately, she began to text Stan when she was feeling down, had questions about issues that arose in therapy sessions, or felt demoralized and wanted to quit therapy. Wanting to establish a working alliance, Stan initially stretched his limits around e-mailing and text messaging and tried to get back to Joanie as quickly as he could. Over time, Joanie's texts and e-mails increased, and Stan began to feel stressed and resentful that Joanie seemed to expect him to be available at all times. He started delaying his response to texts and e-mails in order to get out of having to provide quick or immediate responses. Joanie felt hurt and confused at Stan's newly delayed responses, as this was a substantial change from their initial pattern of communication—a change that Stan had not warned her about. Both Stan and Joanie began to feel frustrated with one another, and when Stan finally brought up the problems associated with texting and e-mailing, Joanie was already angry and confused and felt that Stan had "led her on" by being so available and then just changed gears without saying anything. Fortunately, Stan and Joanie had a very productive heart-to-heart discussion, and Joanie agreed to stop e-mailing and texting and began to call instead. She slipped up a few times and texted or e-mailed, but Stan had told her ahead of time that he wouldn't respond in these circumstance, so she wasn't surprised or hurt when she didn't receive a reply from him. Toward the end of therapy, she told Stan that she was glad they had changed things, as she found their phone calls more helpful than the e-mails and texts they had exchanged early in therapy.

Although it worked out well for Stan and Joanie in the end, Stan could have avoided significant problems if he had clearly oriented Joanie to his policy and limits around electronic communication much earlier in therapy. As mentioned in Chapter 2, electronic communication has become the norm for many people. As such, this norm might enter therapy unless the clinician delineates her or his limits regarding electronic communication ahead of time and conveys these limits to the client. Given the ethical issues associated with electronic communication (e.g., confidentiality risks, the risk that the clinician may receive a text or e-mail communicating suicide intent), clear orientation to any general electronic communication policy also should be part of initial, written informed consent to treatment. I have included an example in Box 3.1.

The clinician should indicate whether she or he is willing to take e-mails or texts and for what purpose. If the clinician is willing to engage in e-mail or texting for skills coaching, this should be made clear to the client, along with the attendant confidentiality risks of sharing sensitive personal information in this manner. Clinicians who are willing to use e-mail or texting for skills coaching can prevent future problems by making it clear that e-mail or text coaching, just like phone coaching, must be brief and focused on skills.

Clients sometimes send e-mails or texts conveying suicidal ideation or intent. In these cases, the clinician may feel compelled to respond right away, potentially reinforcing suicidal communication. Also, this situation can raise concerns about liability, as there is now a written example of suicidal communication and potential risk. Therefore, as illustrated in Box 3.1, I tell clients not to share suicidal ideation or intent over e-mail or text. I also let them know that if they do so, and I believe they are at imminent risk, I will contact the police and request a welfare check.

BOX 3.1. Example Electronic Communication Policy

Electronic communication raises several issues. (1) You should be aware that there are risks to the confidentiality of information shared via electronic communication methods, including e-mail, text messaging, social media, and other forms of electronic communication. None of these methods is considered "secure"; thus, confidential information you share electronically could be viewed by unauthorized persons. (2) Electronic communication should not be a substitute for phone contact if you need skills coaching. I believe that I provide better-quality help and skills coaching over the phone, compared with over e-mail or text messaging. (3) It is easy to misinterpret the tone, intent, or demeanor of electronic communication. E-mailing and texting do not capture voice tone, facial expressions, or other interpersonal cues that might help us understand each other and communicate effectively. (4) E-mail communication should not be used in an emergency or to request urgent skills coaching. I receive 200–400 e-mails per week and have limited time to read or respond to individual e-mails; thus, I am not able to read every e-mail or reply right away. Also, if you text or e-mail me and express suicidal thoughts or intent to harm yourself or others, and I think you're at imminent risk of harming yourself or others, I will contact the police and request that they check on your welfare.

Because of many of the concerns I have described above, I discourage the use of e-mail or text messaging to share any personal information (information about your treatment, mental health concerns, history, etc.) or to request help. I will not respond to texts or e-mails about clinical matters (requests for help, skills coaching, disclosure of personal information, emergencies, etc.). Please call me about these issues, or raise them at your next therapy appointment. I only use texting for scheduling purposes, such as if you are running late, would like to confirm your appointment, or would like to know if I'm available at another time. I do *not,* however, use text messaging for cancellations of appointments (you must call me to cancel). As communication via social media (Facebook, Twitter, etc.) poses substantial risks to confidentiality and could compromise our professional relationship, I will not view or respond to communication via social media. Finally, according to ethical and professional guidelines for my profession, any electronic or other communication (e.g., letters, faxes) will be considered part of your clinical file and stored accordingly.

Although some clinicians find e-mailing very useful, I caution clinicians against getting into the pattern where the client shares information over e-mail or text information that could be shared in session. We once saw a client who regularly sent her clinician lengthy e-mails about present or past issues or concerns that she wished to speak about in therapy sessions. Reviewing these e-mails took a significant amount of time, and it was never entirely clear (even after assessing this issue with the client) as to how to use the content of the e-mails productively in session. It appeared that one function of the e-mails was for someone to know what the client was going through, and she had some difficulty expressing herself in session (due to shame and anxiety). Our team advised the clinician to have the client keep a diary between sessions, to bring this diary to sessions, and to spend 5–10 minutes reviewing it together. The client did this, but eventually the diary plan petered out as the client became more comfortable discussing important issues in person.

As many people use social networking applications as a substitute for e-mail, it is important to discuss the role (or lack thereof) of social networking in therapy. To safeguard confidentiality, I recommend that clinicians ask clients to avoid requesting that their clinician be a "friend" on Facebook or any other social networking site. I also caution clients in group treatment to avoid interacting with each other over social media out of concern that they may inadvertently reveal to their many other social media connections how they know the other client(s).

Clarify Expectations Regarding the Client and the Clinician

Other helpful orientation points have to do with what the clinician expects of the client. Generally, it is helpful to expect the client to try alternative skills before calling the clinician. Calling the clinician is one skill, but DBT includes dozens of behavioral skills (Linehan, 2015), and standard CBT includes many others. Early in therapy, some clients have yet to learn many of the skills they need to navigate challenging everyday situations. I try to teach my clients a few distress tolerance skills in the first couple of sessions, usually before orienting them to phone coaching. As a result, I can expect them to have tried some skills before they call. In fact, when a client calls, I almost always ask what other skills she has tried already. If she hasn't tried any skills, I ask her to go and look in her skills binder, identify some helpful skills, try them out, and call me back if needed. It can also be helpful to convey that the clinician expects the client to be open to her or his advice, willing to try new skills, and willing to work with the clinician to minimize or reduce suicide risk (should that topic arise during the call).

The client should also know what to expect of the clinician. During telephone consultation, the clinician will use many of the core principles and related strategies that comprise standard DBT, such as validation, assessment, problem solving, commitment, troubleshooting, and dialectical strategies. The difference is that the clinician is likely to be more directive, briefer, and to the point, and to spend less time assessing or validating, compared with regular therapy sessions. The clinician might seem a little more matter of fact or "business-like" on the phone than she or he does in therapy sessions. If so, it can be helpful to let clients know this ahead of time. One of my students, for example, was seeing a client who called quite regularly. She typically answered the phone and asked him, "How can I help you?" The client was particularly sensitive to interpersonal rejection and felt hurt, thinking the clinician was treating him like a business client and not like someone who has opened up and shared his history and emotional vulnerabilities. He also felt rushed and wanted more time to talk. When they discussed this issue in a future session, the clinician clarified that she is trying to be quick and efficient on the phone, time is short, and the primary goal is to help him tolerate or manage his emotions. This conversation helped the client better understand the style and focus of the calls and tolerate the clinician's style and the limited time to talk. The clinician also realized she was being a little too business-like and tried to strike a more dialectical balance of warmth and efficiency.

Prevent and Manage Initial Challenges in Phone Coaching

The orientation phase also is an important time to assess and solve or prevent problems that might arise in phone coaching. As a starting point, it's helpful to assess the client's previous experiences in phone coaching, troubleshoot, and plan to prevent the reemergence of any previous problems. Orientation regarding how the clinician and client will work together to manage therapy-interfering issues also can be very helpful; I discuss this type of orientation in more detail in Chapter 8. In addition, I recommend that clinicians be prepared to manage a couple of common problems occurring during the beginning of phone coaching: client reluctance to use phone coaching and initial overuse of phone coaching.

Assessing Prior Experiences and Troubleshooting Problems with Phone Coaching

Some clients may have had some experience with phone coaching or regular phone (or electronic) communication with their previous clinicians. Just as it can be helpful early in therapy to assess the client's previous experiences with therapy, it can also be useful to assess and discuss previous experiences with between-session communication. Some clients may have had limited between-session communication focusing primarily on scheduling, whereas others may have had formal DBT phone coaching. Understanding any problems that arose in previous work can help the clinician and client plan to prevent these problems from repeating. Some helpful questions to ask clients about previous phone coaching include the following:

- "Have you ever had regular communication with previous clinicians between sessions?"
- "Have you ever had DBT-oriented phone coaching (often called 'telephone consultation')?"
- "How has this communication generally occurred? By phone, text, e-mail, or other methods?"
- "How often have you communicated with previous clinicians between sessions?"
- "What did you find most helpful about communicating with your clinician between sessions/phone coaching?"
- "Did you find anything unhelpful about such communication/ phone coaching?"
- "Have you ever had any problems with communication with your clinician between sessions?"

Sigrid, for example, asked her new client, Juanita, some of these questions and discovered that Juanita had been in daily contact with the previous clinician by phone and addressed therapy issues via e-mail several times per week. Juanita said that she found this communication helpful because she had a limited social network and was often lonely. She also said she had a difficult time when her therapist went on vacation and felt uncomfortable going more than a few days without a phone call. Knowing this, Sigrid realized she would need to clearly orient Juanita to her approach to phone coaching. She explained that her limits might be different than those of the previous clinician, and that it's possible she won't be as available. She also explained that she doesn't use e-mail for therapy purposes. Furthermore, she explained that calls for support to alleviate loneliness usually are not consistent with the purposes of phone coaching. When Juanita expressed worry that she might have a hard time with this new approach, Sigrid validated her concerns ("It makes sense that you'd be anxious or worried, as this is different from what you're used to, and you came to rely on your clinician's support throughout the week"). She also suggested skills Juanita could use to tolerate these differences and manage loneliness, and over time they worked on ways for Juanita to expand her social support network.

Helping Clients Who Are Initially Reluctant to Use Phone Coaching

Contrary to the concern that clients will overuse phone coaching, I have found that it is much more common for clients to be reluctant to call their clinicians. Many of the clients I have seen have been reluctant to call me out of concern that they will bother me or that I'm too busy to take their calls. Additional common reasons not to call include difficulty asking for help, shame and related reluctance to reveal certain problems, difficulty knowing what to say on the phone, a lack of interpersonal skills needed to effectively ask for help, and worries, anxiety, or fears about talking to the clinician (e.g., that the client won't know what to say, or that the therapist will be annoyed and judge them). Now, some clinicians might breathe a sigh of relief when they hear that their clients are reluctant to place a call. Perhaps you are thinking this is totally fine. We have bigger fish to fry in therapy than helping the client call me when he needs help. For the purpose of this section, however, let's assume that the clinician actually wants to use phone coaching and believes in the value of this method to enhance the generalization of treatment effects.

There are several ways to facilitate the client's early use of phone coaching. All of these methods, however, rely on an assessment of the client's difficulties or reluctance to call. Astute therapeutic questions, in combination with an informal functional (or "chain") analysis, can be an excellent way to start. An example is shown in the dialogue below.

THERAPIST: So, what do you think about giving me a call for one of those three reasons?

CLIENT: I can see why it would help. I want to say that I can do this, but I'm just not sure I can call you.

THERAPIST: Oh, what makes you think that?

CLIENT: Well . . . I don't know. I guess I'm afraid I'd be bothering you. I know you're busy, and you have a family and everything. I don't want to take up your time.

THERAPIST: I see. Are you afraid that I'll be too busy to talk with you, or that I'll be too busy to want to talk with you?

CLIENT: I guess it's more that last part. Too busy to want to talk with me. You're already helping me here. Why would you want to take your personal time away from your family to talk with me?

THERAPIST: OK, I think I get where you're coming from. Like, all this talk about phone coaching is just talk on my part, but I really don't actually want to do it?

CLIENT: Well, when you put it that way . . .

THERAPIST: Right, I can assure you that I'd tell you if I were not willing to do this. I wouldn't have offered it in the first place. And I can see how you might feel some reluctance, and I appreciate your concern about bothering me. In any relationship, it's always helpful to think of the other person's needs, and you seem to do that pretty naturally. Maybe a little too much, though?

CLIENT: Yeah, like we've talked about, I sort of put my needs aside. I'm the one who always asks what other people want to do when we're going out, and I don't really like putting people out.

THERAPIST: Yes, I remember talking about that. We might want to work on that and maybe help you get more balance in your friendships. For now, though, what emotions come up when you think of calling me?

CLIENT: Kind of uncomfortable. I don't know what it is, maybe nervous.

THERAPIST: Sounds a bit like anxiety. Does that fit?

CLIENT: Yeah, I guess I'm anxious about calling. I'm worried you don't really want to help me, and you'll just be annoyed with me for calling.

THERAPIST: OK, I think we're getting clear on what the problem is. You're afraid that I'll be put out and annoyed with you. You know, that's a pretty common fear. And, it's true, I am very busy. Here's the thing: As I mentioned, I agreed to this because I think it's going to help you a lot, and I am willing to take time to do it. How about we agree that, if it seems like you're calling more than I can fit in, I'll let you know, and we'll find some way to make phone coaching work better for both of us.

CLIENT: I think that would be good. It would probably be hard for me to hear, though.

THERAPIST: That might be true, but I've had to have those kinds of conversations many times before, and I'm pretty good at it. I also tend to bring these things up before I become annoyed, so chances are I'll do that with you, too. If you have a hard time talking about it, I can help you through that, too. Agreeing to all of this is one thing, though. It's another thing to do it.

CLIENT: Right, I'm still not so sure.

THERAPIST: OK, here's what I think we should do. You're afraid of calling because you think something bad is going to happen, like me being annoyed with you. But you probably know intellectually that the fear is not likely to come true. I'm not likely to resent you for calling me and get all annoyed with you. When your fear is not likely to come true, the best thing to do is to do what you're afraid of. It's kind of like, if you were afraid of going outside even though there's no danger involved in stepping out your door. The best way for your brain to learn is that there's no danger in stepping out that door. This is a lot like a skill you'll learn later on called "opposite action." The good news is that, because you shared your concerns about calling me, you'll get a jumpstart with this skill.

CLIENT: OK, that makes sense. What would we do, then?

THERAPIST: How about we start with you calling me about 15 minutes

after our session is over? I'm available for a quick call then. We can
get the ball rolling, give you a chance to see what it's like to call, and
hopefully help you learn that it's not so bad.

In the example above, the clinician briefly assessed factors contributing
to the client's reluctance to call. The client was afraid of the clinician's
reaction (e.g., annoyance at being bothered or having to take time to talk
to the client). Once this barrier to calling was clear, a solution involving
exposure and opposite-action-oriented principles and skills seemed most
appropriate. The clinician used the dialectical strategy of "making lem-
onade out of lemons" (Linehan, 1993a) by saying that the client's reluctance to call will give her a jumpstart with an important skill (opposite
action).

Another approach is to use irreverence or other DBT strategies to
address this situation. Irreverence in DBT is a therapeutic style involving
the therapist making unexpected remarks, using humour, being matter-
of-fact about outrageous topics, directly and intensely confronting the client's behavior, and so forth (Linehan, 1993a). This type of approach can
be used strategically to help the client understand the implications of his
or her behavior, get the client's attention, or help him or her think about
the situation differently (Lynch, Chapman, Kuo, Rosenthal, & Linehan,
2006). If a suicidal client, for example, was reluctant to take up his clinician's time, the clinician might state that he would rather hear from the
client at 10:00 P.M. than from the hospital at 3:00 A.M.

In some cases, the client might not have developed the interpersonal
skills to effectively ask for help. In this case, it would be useful for the
clinician to use the principles of skills training and coaching discussed
in Chapter 5 to help the client learn how to effectively ask for help on
the phone. I have often found that a helpful initial step with clients who
aren't sure what to say or how to ask for help on the phone is to simply
coach them to call and say, "Hi Dr. Chapman, it's Sally." I let them know
that's all they really need to say, and that I'll take charge from there. Over
time, of course, I'd expect them to say more and take a more active role.
Through shaping and regular practice, clients often learn how to effectively ask for what they need. Furthermore, learning how to ask for help
in the context of phone coaching will ideally generalize to other areas
where it could be useful to ask for help and support.

If the problem contributing to reluctance to call is an emotion such as
shame, interventions focusing on acceptance, mindfulness, and opposite

action can be quite helpful. A client, for example, who feels ashamed of his problems may benefit from (1) practicing mindful observation of the experience of shame and (2) engaging in opposite action by reversing the action tendencies associated with shame, such as by sitting up straight, making eye contact, and directly talking about his problems. This work might first occur in session, and then the clinician might help the client to engage in similar behaviors during coaching calls. The client, for example, might work on openly disclosing topics he feels ashamed about, speaking in a direct and forthright manner, and changing his posture (even though the therapist will not get to view this change).

Helping Clients Who Initially Overuse Phone Coaching

At times, clients start off by calling (or e-mailing, texting, and using other forms of electronic messaging) the clinician too often. Clients may initially overuse phone coaching for a variety of reasons. Complex clients with multiple problem areas may be in crisis at the beginning of treatment, requiring help to stay safe and get through a difficult situation. Other clients might lack social support or need help to get through everyday life difficulties, and there has not yet been enough time to teach the client skills to establish other supports or navigate everyday problems more independently. Some clients have had previous clinicians with broader limits who were more available than the current clinician wishes to be (as mentioned above with Bob and Sally, and Sigrid and Juanita). Clients also might overuse phone coaching because they wish to establish a connection with the clinician, are testing out whether they can work with the clinician, or simply have many questions or concerns to address.

Effectively managing this situation requires a clear assessment of the factors contributing to the client's calling, the function of client calls (e.g., to regulate emotions, to alleviate loneliness, to test the clinician), any related skill deficits, emotions, or cognitions, and so on. I strongly urge clinicians to intervene early to avoid stepping onto the path to burnout. To do this, I recommend some of the observing-limits strategies discussed in Chapter 8 and elaborated in Linehan (1993a) and elsewhere (Chapman & Rosenthal, 2016). Briefly, I recommend that clinicians broach this topic in a clear, behaviorally specific, and nonjudgmental manner as soon as they notice that clients are calling too often. I also recommend that clinicians (1) clarify why it is important to address frequent calling, (2) convey the message that these type of discussions are normal and to be expected from time to time, and (3) work with the client to reduce the calls while helping her meet her needs through other means. A brief example is described below:

> "Today, I'd like to start off by talking about how our phone calls have been going. We've been working together for a few weeks now, and I've noticed that you've been calling me daily (and sometimes more than once a day) over the past couple of weeks. Much of the time, when you call, it seems like you're really having a hard time, so I can understand why you need my help. As we've discussed, these calls are to help you learn to use skills in your everyday life, and I know it has been hard not knowing many of the skills. So, it makes sense to me that you've been reaching out, and at the same time I know I won't be able to keep fitting in daily calls. Given all of my other work and personal commitments, I'm finding it hard to carve out the time to talk with you this often, and I don't want phone coaching to become a stressor on our work. I also want to make sure I stay willing to do the phone calls, and if there are too many, my willingness is going to go down. Let's see if we can talk a little less often and make it easier for you to get the support you need from other people. I'm interested in your thoughts about how phone coaching is going, too, so I'd like us to talk about that and find a way to make sure it works well for both of us."

Being Dialectical about Orientation

Orientation is inherently a dialectical process. Orientation prevents problems and makes phone coaching more effective. With a clear road map to phone coaching, clients are much more able to navigate it in a way that works best for them and the clinician. Orientation, however, can easily devolve into rigid rule following and limit setting, which, as discussed earlier, are inconsistent with DBT principles. It's not possible to prevent all problems or orient the client to all possible aspects of phone coaching. A synthesis in this dialectic is to provide orientation at the beginning and then to continue to orient and reorient and observe limits consistently as phone coaching unfolds. Orientation, as mentioned, does not just occur at the beginning of a given treatment or treatment modality but often is used throughout treatment to emphasize the focus of a phone coaching call (skills coaching); the plan, structure, and agenda for each call (discussed in Chapter 4); and so forth. Therefore, orientation in DBT phone coaching is much like setting forth a hiking route and plan at the beginning of the journey and remaining responsive to shifting weather and terrain, continuing to provide orientation and guiding the client throughout.

Summary

In summary, clear and thorough orientation can help pave the way for effective phone coaching. Ideally, during orientation, the clinician distinguishes phone coaching from therapy, provides a clear rationale for this mode of intervention, and provides guidance regarding when and why to call. Regarding the latter, there are generally three key reasons to call: (1) for help with skills coaching, (2) for issues in the therapy relationship, and (3) for emergencies or crises. It is also helpful to orient the client regarding the brief nature of phone coaching calls. Orientation should thoroughly address any clinician limits around phone coaching or electronic communication methods, as well as expectations regarding client or clinician behavior during phone coaching. For another excellent discussion of orientation to phone coaching, consistent with many of the guidelines in this chapter, see Ben-Porath (2015).

There also are several ways to prevent or manage initial challenges in phone coaching. It can be helpful to assess the client's prior experiences with phone coaching and determine whether there are any problems to solve or prevent. One common challenges during the beginning phase of phone coaching is client reluctance to call the clinician. In this case, it can be helpful to assess barriers to calling, engage in collaborative problem solving, and encourage the client to practice calling. Another common challenge is that the client might call too often in the beginning of therapy. To manage this situation, it is helpful to catch it early, bring it up with the client, and work together to make phone coaching work best for both parties.

CHAPTER 4

Navigating and Structuring Phone Coaching Calls

The focus of this chapter is on strategies to effectively structure phone coaching calls. I start by discussing how to organize time during phone coaching calls, using DBT targeting principles. Next, I offer a discussion of how to effectively manage contingencies in a way that supports effective phone coaching. Much of the rest of the chapter has to do with how to structure the beginning, middle, and ending portions of the phone coaching call, and how the 24-hour rule may change this structure. As this structure is not described in the original DBT manual (Linehan, 1993a), what I outline in this chapter comes from years of experience with phone coaching, training and supervision with Marsha Linehan, discussions of phone coaching with other DBT colleagues, and examples and advice from outstanding co-trainers I have worked with while giving workshops and trainings on DBT. It can be useful to regularly debrief phone coaching at the next therapy session; thus, I have included some guidance on this topic. Finally, I present a discussion of dialectical principles applied to structuring.

Organizing Time during Phone Coaching

The DBT principle of *targeting* guides the amount of time and effort spent on particular topics during therapy. The clinician uses a hierarchy of treatment targets that largely determines the amount of session resources (time, effort, etc.) devoted to certain topics, corresponding to different categories of client behavior. The different categories include (1) life-threatening behavior, (2) therapy-destroying behavior, (3) therapy-interfering behavior, (4) quality-of-life interfering behavior, (5) skills deficits, and (6) secondary targets.

Life-threatening behavior includes any behavior involving the deliberate, acute infliction of damage to oneself or others, including suicide attempts, nonsuicidal self-injury, and aggressive or violent behavior toward others. Also included are suicidal threats or crises; plans or preparation for suicide, self-injury, or harm to someone else. Not typically included are behaviors that may be self-damaging over the long run, such as substance use, disordered eating, reckless driving, or other impulsive, potentially self-damaging behaviors, where the damage is not acute or intentional. In phone coaching, life-threatening behavior is given highest importance. If the client is at imminent risk of suicide or self-injury, the clinician will devote the majority of phone coaching time to the assessment and management of risk and skills the client can use to reduce risk. In Chapter 7, I describe strategies for calls focused on crises and suicide risk.

Therapy-destroying behavior involves any behavior that makes it impossible to continue therapy in a safe and effective manner, such as physical aggression or threats of violence toward the clinician, staff, or other clients; stalking; vandalism; theft; unusual or outrageous sexual behaviors, among other possibilities. Therapy-destroying behavior during phone coaching normally takes the form of a highly hostile attitude, threats, severe and unrelenting criticism, or overwhelmingly frequent, intense, or lengthy communication.

Therapy-interfering behavior is any behavior on the part of the clinician or client that (1) makes it difficult to implement treatment, (2) creates problems in the therapy relationship, or (3) hampers the client's progress toward his or her goals. Common examples in phone coaching include the client calling too frequently; not returning calls; being disrespectful, hostile, or uncommunicative; calling for reasons unrelated to skills coaching; and unwillingness to discuss or try skills. Common examples of clinician behaviors include failing to return calls; being disrespectful or judgmental; failing to appropriately structure calls; calling in a nonconfidential setting; calling when inebriated, distracted (e.g., when driving), or otherwise indisposed; or engaging in individual therapy on the phone.

Quality-of-life interfering behavior includes behaviors or conditions that hamper the client's ability to reach important goals and establish a desired quality of life. Common examples include symptoms or disorders impeding functioning (e.g., depression, psychosis, severe anxiety, substance use problem, eating disorders, severe interpersonal dysfunction, and functional impairments (lack of employment or home, financial destitution, social alienation). Situations interfering with the client's quality of life (e.g., interpersonal conflict, daily life stressors and hassles, losses, changes in living environment) usually prompt phone coaching calls. Phone coaching emphasizes skills the client can use to cope with these situations and only focuses on solving the client's most immediate and short-term quality-of-life problems. For example, a client might lack consistent social support and has called for help with loneliness. The clinician would coach the client on how to cope with loneliness in the short term (e.g., that particular evening, or the next couple of days). Individual therapy sessions would help improve the client's social support and reduce loneliness over the long run.

Skill deficits include the lack of behavioral skills needed for the client to improve his or her life and work toward achieving important goals. The four main skill domains in DBT include mindfulness, interpersonal effectiveness, emotion regulation, and distress tolerance. The client may have deficits in these or other areas, such as organization, self-management, employment, generic social skills, or other domains. Phone coaching focuses on generalizing skills the client is learning in therapy rather than on teaching the client new skills. The expectation is that the client will learn behavioral skills over the longer run in a DBT or other skills-focused group and, as needed, in individual therapy. At times, however, phone coaching might involve brief teaching on practical skills that are easy to implement. One example might include brief teaching on the skills of distraction or self-soothing, which are easy to learn and implement right away.

Secondary targets include "dialectical dilemmas" (Linehan, 1993a), which are polarized behavioral patterns that sometimes occur in the treatment of patients with BPD or other complex disorders. One example is the polarity of *active passivity* versus *apparent competence*, whereby the patient vacillates between appearing competent and able to cope with his problems and function well despite the presence of severe dysfunction (apparent competence), and actively recruiting others to meet his needs (active passivity). Apparent competence occurs when the clinician believes the client needs less help and support than he actually needs, whereas active passivity often results in the clinician and others taking a much more active role than usual or preferable to help meet the client's needs. Among the dialectical dilemmas, this is perhaps the one most relevant to phone coaching. When apparent competence during phone coaching belies the client's desperate need for help, the clinician may not take appropriate actions to provide adequate help or address the client's suicide risk. When the client engages in active passivity with regard to phone coaching (often showing up as repeated calls, e-mails, texts, and urgent requests for assistance), the clinician may work much harder than the client, extend his limits to provide an unusual amount of help, and end up on the path to burnout.

As displayed in Table 4.1, the different DBT modes have different target hierarchies, depending on the role of the clinician in each mode. In phone coaching, the clinician's role is to guide the client in the use of skills in everyday life. With the exception of times when life-threatening behavior is imminent, the clinician spends most of each phone call help-ing the client use skills in her everyday life. As mentioned in Chapter 1 on reasons for the client to call the clinician, a phone coaching call might also address the client's sense of alienation, conflict, or disconnectedness from the clinician. These relationship-focused calls, however, often focus on skills the client can use to tolerate or regulate emotions related to his relationship concerns.

When the clinician has this hierarchy of targets in mind, phone coaching is more likely to go smoothly and effectively. This is why I rec-ommend below that the clinician and client come up with a brief agenda at the beginning of the call. That way, the clinician can organize the

TABLE 4.1. Target Hierarchies for Different DBT Modes

Individual therapy	Group skills training	Phone coaching
• Life-threatening behavior	• Therapy-destroying behavior	• Life-threatening behavior
• Therapy-destroying or -interfering behavior	• Skill deficits	• Skill generalization
• Quality-of-life interfering behavior	• Therapy-interfering behavior	• Sense of alienation from clinician
• Skill deficits		
• Secondary targets (dialectical dilemmas)		

topics to be addressed according to the hierarchy and decide what to focus on. If the client, for example, calls and says she needs help with interpersonal skills to apologize for yelling at her partner, but she also reports high suicidal intent and planning, the therapist might table discussions of the relationship issue, focusing instead on skills to reduce suicide risk.

Effectively Managing Contingencies during Phone Coaching

I further discuss contingency management to manage problems arising in phone coaching in Chapter 8. Here, I remind the reader of the importance of contingency management as a tool to maintain the structure and focus of phone coaching calls. The clinician must be attentive to the type of behavior in which the client is engaging. Is the client engaging in behavior that facilitates phone coaching or takes it off-track? During phone coaching calls, some potential client behaviors to maintain or increase include discussing skills, remaining on topic, expressing willingness or commitment to use the skills discussed, providing a brief and useful description of the problem prompting the call, responding to the clinician's questions or comments, and collaborative problem solving. Behaviors to decrease include the client making off-topic statements, engaging in noncollaborative behaviors, expressing unwillingness to discuss or use skills, venting, remaining silent or nonresponsive, and expressing hostility toward the clinician.

If the client is engaging in one of the above behaviors, to increase a positive behavior, the clinician might consider ways to differentially reinforce those behaviors (i.e., by using differential reinforcement of other or alternative behaviors; Farmer & Chapman, 2008, 2016). Potential reinforcers could include increased warmth or responsivity, more attention, validation, and genuine expressions of caring and support on the part of the clinician. Other reinforcers could include the clinician providing a slightly longer call (if contact with the clinician is a positive reinforcer) or a slightly shorter call (if reductions in time spent with the clinician is a negative reinforcer). One of my previous clients, for example, had tremendous difficulty calling me. He found the act of seeking help and talking to me about his problems on the phone to be embarrassing and shameful. While we worked on overcoming this problem over time, in the short term spending less time with me on the phone seemed to negatively reinforce effective behavior. As a result, I tried to get down to business and get off the phone much more quickly when the client engaged in behavior that facilitated our phone coaching calls.

If the client is engaging in behaviors that take phone coaching off-track, the clinician should avoid reinforcing those behaviors. The clinician could ignore or block the behaviors by consistently redirecting the client or by withdrawing warmth or responsivity (e.g., speaking in a more matter-of-fact, down-to-business voice tone). Although aversive consequences (i.e., punishment) are used sparingly in DBT, common strategies include shortening or ending calls with clients who are unwilling to discuss skills, expressing disapproval (e.g., if the client is being hostile), and directly confronting the client's behavior (Chapman & Rosenthal, 2016; Linehan, 1993a). The effective use of contingency management strategies can go a long way in facilitating the structuring of phone calls. To use these strategies, the clinician must remain mindful of the type of behavior the client is engaging in and compassionately focus on what is best for the client during each particular call.

Structuring Phone Coaching Calls

Structure is a common and core feature of both CBT and DBT. Individual and group DBT and CBT sessions often are structured according to a schedule of activities occurring at the beginning, middle, and end of the session. Within this structure, there is flexibility to accommodate the individual client's needs and preferences and to address emergent issues. The structuring of therapy activities facilitates efficient work on targets that are relevant to the client's goals.

Phone coaching calls often tend to have a particular structure or flow of activities. Structure is arguably even more critical in phone coaching than in individual or group sessions, given the limited time available to coach the client in skills. Individual or group sessions might last 1–2 hours, whereas phone coaching ideally lasts from less than 5 to 10 or 15 minutes. That is not much time to get important work done. Therefore, to maximize the effectiveness of phone coaching, it is important for the clinician to structure his or her calls and make the most efficient use of the time available.

Structure also can help focus and regulate clients experiencing high levels of distress. Such clients often have difficulty organizing their thoughts and planning through which skills to use or how to use them. I often have observed that a structured and organized phone coaching call seems to help clients focus and organize their thoughts and can have a soothing or regulating effect.

The Beginning Portion of a Phone Coaching Call

It can be helpful to divide coaching calls into the beginning, the middle, and the ending portion of the calls. (See Table 4.2 for a brief summary of the structure of phone coaching calls and helpful tips and pointers for the beginning, middle, and ending portions of these calls.) The clinician can set the stage for an effective phone coaching call by structuring the call from the beginning. Briefly orienting the client to the nature of the call can clarify what the ensuing conversation will (and will not) focus on. It is also helpful to elicit a brief summary of the problem prompting

TABLE 4.2. The Structure of Phone Coaching Calls

Portion	Goals	Tips
Beginning	Quickly assess and understand the problem.	• Briefly orient the client to the purpose and logistics (e.g., time available) for the call. • Ask for a brief summary of the problem. • Focus on emotions. • Convey the focus on skills. • Convey the expectation that the client has tried skills already. • Use the hierarchy of targets to organize time. • Manage contingencies effectively.
Middle	Coach the client in the effective use of skills (typically to tolerate or regulate emotions).	• Use effective coaching strategies (see Chapters 4 and 5). • Structure the flow of the discussion. • Use contingency-management strategies as needed. • Keep the focus on skills coaching.
End	Help the client move forward with an effective plan to use skills.	• Briefly summarize the discussion and skills plan. • If needed, use commitment strategies, troubleshoot potential barriers, and/or plan for follow-up.

the call and to place emphasis on the client's emotional experience and use of skills to regulate or tolerate emotions. I also recommend that clinicians convey the expectation that clients already have tried such skills by routinely asking what they've tried before calling the clinician. Finally, it can be helpful and is often critical (in the case of suicide risk) to keep the phone coaching target hierarchy (discussed above) in mind at the beginning and throughout the call. I expand on and provide examples of these points and key beginning strategies below.

Provide Brief Orientation

One of the first basic steps for any phone coaching call is to provide a brief orientation. Even if the clinician has already provided a thorough orientation at the beginning of treatment (see Chapter 3), it is still helpful to reorient the client at the beginning of each phone coaching call. This orientation may occur either before or after the clinician assesses the problem prompting the call. Ideally, orientation should address the focus of the call and any relevant logistics, such as how much time is available. One example of this type of brief orientation is shown below:

> "I'm glad you called me for help with this problem. So, we've got about 10 minutes. Let's make sure we use our time well. We're going to focus mainly on the types of skills that might help you through this situation. Our main goal is to help you regulate or tolerate your emotions over the next little while. Hopefully, we'll be able to come up with a good plan."

In this example, the clinician reminds the client of how much time is available and of the importance of being efficient. Clients often initially approach calls as if they are open-ended, lengthy discussions. A clear time limit conveys the message that the client and the clinician must be efficient and get to work quickly. Consider how diligently you would study if an exam was coming up in 2 days versus 2 months. What if the deadline was open-ended and you could take the exam whenever you felt like it? How much do you think you would work on a day-to-day basis? Goal-setting theory (and everyday common sense) suggests that awareness of time limits facilitates efficient work (Locke & Latham, 2002; Lunenberg, 2011). While it is not always necessary to specify a time limit to the client, the client needs to understand that time is limited.

The clinician also emphasized skills. Reminding the client of the focus on skills can help prevent phone coaching calls from turning into therapy sessions. For the caller, it can be easy to slip into the role of a client in an hour-long therapy session, where the focus is on longer-term goals. Clients sometimes call to seek the kind of help (e.g., solving relationship problems) that would be best suited for a therapy session. At other times, clients may call to alleviate loneliness, get something off their chest, or to use the clinician as a sounding board. Orientation should clarify that these issues will not be the focus of the call, and if the call veers in these directions, the therapist should steer it back to skills coaching.

Briefly Assess the Problem Prompting the Call

It is helpful for the clinician to get at least a general sense of the problem prompting the call. Typically, skills coaching will target emotions, thoughts, and actions related to this problem; thus, the clinician's goal is to learn *just enough* about the problem to provide helpful coaching. There is not enough time to assess problems as thoroughly as the clinician might in an individual therapy session; therefore, it is helpful to let the client know that the clinician needs a rough idea of the problem. I often find it helpful to ask the client to provide a brief summary of the problem (e.g., "Please give me just a brief summary of what you're going through so I can figure out how best to help."). Here, the way the clinician asks the client about the problem often can determine whether the client provides a short or extensive version. Please read the questions and prompts below, and consider which ones are most likely to elicit a brief, concise summary:

- "Why don't you take a minute and tell me a little about what's going on?"
- "What kind of problem are you dealing with?"
- "Let's spend a minute or two discussing the problem, and then I'd like to know which skills you've tried so far."
- "Tell me what's happening."
- "OK, so I'd like to hear a brief, *Reader's Digest* version of what you're going through so that I can come up with some helpful suggestions."

- "How are you doing?"
- "What can I help you with?"

From the first, third, and fifth questions, it is fairly clear that the clinician is seeking a brief description of the problem. Furthermore, in some of these examples, the emphasis on skills is clear. In contrast, the second, fourth, sixth, and seventh questions/prompts are too broad and may elicit lengthy descriptions of the problem. This is why I would suggest that clinicians avoid starting off by simply asking the client what is happening, how she or he is doing, and so on. This may seem like a rather obvious point, but when a client calls you in great distress, you can be tempted to avoid structuring the discussion and to simply be present to listen empathetically. Any follow-up questions should focus on the most relevant information and ideally elicit brief responses.

Focus on Emotions

As the goal of phone coaching generally is to help clients figure out how to use skills to regulate or tolerate their emotions in the short term, often the most relevant information has to do with the client's immediate emotional experience. This focus on emotions is also in keeping with the emotion-focused nature of DBT and the biosocial theory emphasizing the role of emotions and emotion regulation in BPD (Crowell et al., 2009; Linehan, 1993a). Even if a clinician is not working with clients who have BPD or is not practicing the DBT approach, he or she will find it helpful to understand the client's specific emotional experience. Different emotional states are sometimes amenable to different types of skills; thus, the clinician should seek information on the specific emotions the client is having the hardest time managing or tolerating. An example dialogue is presented below.

THERAPIST: Why don't you take a minute or so and let me know what you're dealing with, so we can figure out what skills might be most helpful.

CLIENT: Oh, my God, I don't know if I can get through this. I just got a text from my boyfriend that he needs some distance. He wants to take a break for a couple of weeks. He said that the way I've been is just too much for him. This always happens to me! I feel like I'm such a big weight on everybody. What am I going to do if I lose him!

THERAPIST: It can be so hard to hear that kind of thing, and you're thinking you're a burden and will lose him. Can you tell me a little about the emotions coming up for you? I'd like to know about the emotions you're having the hardest time with right now.

CLIENT: I don't know, I just feel so miserable, just awful! I just, I just don't know if I can go on like this without him.

THERAPIST: Right now, the idea of not being close to him feels unbearable. We will figure out a way to help you get through this. We're going to focus on skills to help you ride this out, and then we'll talk more when we meet. When you say "miserable" and "awful," what do you mean?

CLIENT: I don't know, I mean I'm just sick about what happened.

THERAPIST: You've mentioned the thoughts going through your mind, like you're going to lose him, you're a burden, and why do you always do this. I'm wondering what kinds of action urges you're having— like, what you feel like doing . . .

CLIENT: I want to call him and convince him not to do this to us. I don't know, I also just feel like hiding or curling up somewhere and dying.

THERAPIST: OK, so I'm going to make a guess that you're dealing with fear and maybe shame?

CLIENT: That seems pretty close. I'm terrified of losing him. I'm also feeling like it's all my fault, so maybe guilty or ashamed or something. Why do I always do this?

THERAPIST: Nice job describing how you're feeling. I see that this is so painful for you. You're afraid that your reaching out to him has pushed him away—exactly the opposite of what you wanted. Let's try to remember that, so far, he says he wants a break. So, we don't really know if that means it's over or going to be over. For now, let's focus on how to get through what you're feeling. We should also talk about skills for thoughts, like your worry that he'll leave you for good or that you're just a big burden, and that kind of thing. Does that sound good for now?

In this example, the client initially had difficulty labeling her specific emotional states. She presented as overwhelmed and described her emotional experience in vague terms, such as "miserable" and "awful." This is common. Indeed, there is some evidence that people with BPD have difficulty differentiating between similarly valenced emotional states (Suvak et al., 2011; Zaki, Coffman, Rafaeli, Berenson, & Downey, 2013). Even clients who have had training in emotion regulation skills will often describe vague or general emotional states when they are highly distressed.

The clinician first tried to elicit more specific information by simply asking the client what she meant by "miserable" or "awful." This strategy often works, but the client continued to have difficulty coming up with specific emotion names. The clinician then prompted the client to describe action urges related to her emotions. In the DBT framework (Linehan, 1993b, 2015), emotions have many components (discussed further in Chapter 6), including physiological (changes in neurochemistry and other biological activity, bodily sensations, urges to engage in particular actions), behavioral (actions, expression of emotion), and cognitive (thoughts, perceptions, appraisals) components. Particular thoughts, action urges, sensations, and actions can sometimes distinguish different emotional states. As shame often is associated with urges to hide, and Sally mentioned the desire to "hide, curl up, and die," the clinician guessed that Sally might be experiencing shame. It was also clear from her thoughts that she was afraid of losing her boyfriend. Once these specific emotions are clear, the clinician and client can zero-in on potentially helpful skills.

Inquire about Skills the Client Has Tried

Once the clinician understands the problem prompting the call, he or she will find it helpful to ask the client about skills that she or he has already tried to cope with this problem. This question at least indirectly conveys the impression that the clinician expects the client to have tried skills before calling. As mentioned in Chapter 3, I recommend that clinicians orient clients to this expectation at the beginning of therapy. Asking what skills the client has tried also is another way to convey the therapeutic emphasis on skills.

I often try to be less available to clients who call without first trying skills. The client who repeatedly calls without having tried skills is at risk of becoming reliant on phone coaching and may be less likely to generalize skills to everyday life or to life beyond the end of therapy. It also is important to remember that phone coaching involves helping the client with skills he is trying to use. If the client has not been using skills, there is less material for coaching. This situation is akin to a tennis student asking for advice on her serve without showing the instructor how her current serve looks. For these reasons, I often ask clients who say they have not tried skills yet to get off the phone, look in their skills binder, and try out a few skills that seem helpful. At that point, I end the call, and I let the client know he can call me later for help with skills coaching if needed. This is another example of differential reinforcement of alternative behavior (DRA; Farmer & Chapman, 2008, 2016), where reinforcement is provided only if the client engages in certain behaviors. In this case, the client receives the potential positive reinforcer (help from the clinician) only if he has already tried skills. With new clients who are unsure of what type of skills might help, I spend a little time helping them figure out which sets of skills (e.g., distress tolerance vs. interpersonal effectiveness) might help most before asking them to give it a shot.

As with any therapeutic strategy, it is important to apply this contingency in a compassionate and flexible manner that fits the client's specific situation. A client may call in considerable distress about particularly upsetting life events (such as a loved one having passed away, recent assault, or losing a job), having not tried any skills just yet. The client might be so upset and overwhelmed that she has not been able to use skills or might need support, understanding, or encouragement before moving forward with skills. Many people have difficulty asking others for help, often due to emotional (e.g., embarrassment, shame) or cognitive barriers (e.g., perfectionism) or interpersonal skill deficits. Calling the clinician for help could then be considered a skill in itself. In these cases, the clinician might provide help, support, or coaching even if the client has yet to try skills. I recommend, however, that clinicians attend to whether their clients have gotten into a pattern of calling before using skills. I also find it helpful at the beginning of therapy to briefly teach my clients some of the skills from the distress tolerance section focused on how to manage extreme emotions (Linehan, 2015; also summarized in Chapter 6). That way, my clients at least have a few skills to try before calling, and if they can reduce their distress somewhat, phone coaching calls tend to be more effective.

Use the Target Hierarchy to Structure the Call

After assessing the primary problem(s) prompting the call, the clinician should organize time and effort in a manner that is commensurate with the phone coaching target hierarchy. If the client, for example, has called reporting distress regarding a recent conflict with her boyfriend and also is imminently suicidal, the clinician is likely to focus primarily on reducing suicide risk (following guidelines from Chapter 8). In doing so, the clinician will likely coach the client on skills to tolerate emotions or avoid further prompting events for these emotions (e.g., contact or further conflict with the boyfriend). Suicide-specific strategies are likely to take up a significant proportion of the call. In contrast, if the client were not imminently suicidal and called reporting similar problems, the primary focus would likely be on skills she can use to deal with the conflict she reports. This might be a subtle distinction, as both calls would focus on skills, but in the imminent-risk scenario, the priority is to help the client use skills to cope without attempting suicide. In the other scenarios, the primary problem prompting the call is a sense of alienation, disconnection, or distress about the therapy relationship. In these cases, the primary focus would be on skills to help enhance the client's sense of connection with the clinician and/or to regulate and tolerate emotions related to the therapy relationship.

The Middle of a Phone Coaching Call

The middle portion of the call focuses on skills coaching, most often emphasizing skills to help the client regulate or tolerate emotions (but also including any of the skills used in DBT or other evidence-based approaches). Although phone coaching does not generally involve solving life problems that are best addressed in individual therapy, if the client presents a problem that is easy to solve quickly, the clinician might coach the client on how to solve it. The middle section is the meat of the phone coaching call, should take up the largest amount of time, and often involves the use of a variety of DBT treatment strategies (e.g., structural strategies, acceptance, change, validation, problem solving) and stylistic strategies (e.g., irreverence, reciprocity) (Linehan, 1993a), in addition to skills coaching. In this section, I emphasize structural strategies to help the clinician maintain focus on skills coaching.

Structure the Conversation

Clinicians often must take an active and directive role in phone coaching. There is often not enough time for the clinician to use strategies that are commonly employed in individual therapy, such as Socratic questioning (Beck, 1979), motivational interviewing (Miller & Rollnick, 2002, 2012), throwing the ball in the client's court and waiting for her to come up with effective skills or solutions, and so on. Clinicians taking an active and directive role will help make the most efficient use of time during phone coaching. One way to do this is to structure the conversation.

Clinicians can structure the conversation in several ways. As mentioned earlier, *orientation* can help the client to understand what is expected of her or him. Orientation also can help guide the client through the conversation, much like a hiking guide would guide clients through different trails in the forest (e.g., "OK, we're going to stop here for a pitstop and then proceed west for another 45 minutes. Watch out for rattlesnakes."). Orientation might involve providing information on what the clinician and client will talk about, which specific skills to focus on, and why these skills might help. Orientation also involves statements that help direct the flow of the conversation, such as the clinician indicating that it would be helpful to focus the discussion on a particular topic. An example of this use of orientation is presented in the dialogue below:

THERAPIST: OK, so Sally I think we should spend a few minutes talking about skills that will help you get through the fear and shame that you are experiencing. You mentioned that you've already tried distraction, but you're having trouble with that.

CLIENT: Yeah, I mean, sure I can distract myself, but as soon as I stop watching TV or get off the phone with someone, I still feel just as bad as I did before. I just don't know what I'm going to do without him. I can't stand the idea of being alone, and I put so much into this relationship that . . .

THERAPIST: I know, this is so hard. I'm really glad to hear that you've already been trying some skills. And we will definitely have time to talk more about the stuff about your relationship and being alone in our next session. For now, let's come back to what you said about distraction. Let's talk a bit about how distraction works. I think we can also come up with a couple of other skills that would help.

CLIENT: OK.

THERAPIST: Distraction is a short-term skill. It probably won't make you feel better for a long time or solve the problem you're dealing with. It will, however, probably take the edge off during the distracting activity. That's why you often have to stack up your distraction skills, so that you don't have too much time in between. Make sense?

CLIENT: Oh yeah, I remember that from group. It's just so exhausting to keep on trying so hard to cope all the time. It would be so much easier just to give up, give in, and drink or something.

THERAPIST: Absolutely, it might be much easier in the short run but probably harder in the long run. We've talked about the problems drinking causes, right?

CLIENT: I know.

THERAPIST: I don't think you would have called if you weren't willing to keep going and keep trying.

CLIENT: That's true, I do want to keep going.

THERAPIST: Good, so let's come back to ways that you can stack up your distraction skills this evening. Then, I've got some ideas for self-soothing. I also have some thoughts about things that you should probably avoid doing, given how afraid you are of losing your boyfriend.

In this example, the clinician used orientation to guide the conversation. He began by describing what he and Sally will be talking about, namely, skills that would be helpful to get through fear and shame. When Sally began to talk about the broader relationship issue, the clinician briefly validated her concerns, mentioned that he was glad she used her skills, and reminded Sally that they will have time to talk about the broader relationship issue in their next therapy session. The clinician redirected Sally toward a discussion of skills, again using orienting strategies. This combination of validating, redirecting, and orienting can help direct the flow of the conversation without dismissing the client's statements or concerns. Subsequently, the clinician provided Sally with some important information on the way in which distraction works. When Sally indicated that she is having a hard time sustaining effort, the clinician validated this and used orienting statements to let Sally know what they are going to talk about.

Beyond the use of orienting, redirecting, and so on, there is another effective but often unsung therapeutic strategy that can help structure phone coaching conversations. This is the art of interrupting. I would argue that interrupting skillfully, tactfully, and in a way that maintains the therapy relationship is one of the more important skills to use during phone coaching (and assessment/treatment more broadly). Many clinicians have a difficult time interrupting their clients. When I was first learning therapy, being a polite, congenial Canadian, I had an especially hard time with this issue. It wasn't too long before I found myself drowning in lengthy conversations that went nowhere. I needed to learn how to effectively interrupt my clients, and to do this I needed to observe others who are good at it and then get some practice myself. Fortunately, I had good mentors who could interrupt almost anyone, and I learned a few tips from them. I also practiced a fair bit, and I'm not sure my wife appreciated it!

Skillful interrupting requires practice. In our DBT teams and classes, we often have clinicians go around the room and practice interrupting clients who are venting or talking at length about off-topic issues. We've often found that catchphrases that get peoples' attention are particularly effective. I initially learned this from Marsha Linehan, who developed DBT and is incredibly skilled at interrupting. Her most common catchphrase is something like, "OK, dear, here's the thing." This strategy is effective precisely because it gets peoples' attention. When she says this, we're all wondering what the "thing" is, so we stop talking and listen. As an aside, some of us had once scheduled a meeting with Marsha, and she did not know what we were meeting about. She came in, sat down, and said, "OK, here's the thing . . ." and then quickly realized that she did not know what the "thing" was! She still had us quietly listening and waiting for what she might say. I would recommend that clinicians embarking on phone coaching gain some practice at interrupting their clients skillfully, and that they develop such catchphrases of their own (or steal good ones from others). I'd even go so far as to say that, if you don't learn to interrupt, validate, redirect, and orient during phone coaching, you're doomed.

Structuring the Ending Segment of the Call

The primary goal of the ending portion of the skills training call is to help the client move forward with an effective plan to use his or her skills. Discussions generally focus on the plan that the client and clinician have devised, the client's commitment to this plan, and any factors that might get in the way (i.e., troubleshooting). Just as brief orientation can be helpful in the beginning and middle of the coaching call, orientation can also help structure the ending segment of the call. For example, once Sally and her clinician have come up with a viable plan to use skills, the clinician might say something like the following:

> I feel good about this plan. I'm looking forward to talking with you more in our next session. Now, before we finish up, I'd like to spend a minute or two making sure you're on board with this whole thing and briefly discussing anything that might get in the way."

Often, if there is enough time available, it is helpful for the clinician to briefly summarize and check in with the client on her or his level of commitment to implement the plan:

> "So, our plan is for you to go home and call Jenny. After you talk with Jenny, you're going to watch the *Big Bang Theory*, take a bath for about half an hour, and get ready for bed. Our plan is also for you to avoid calling, texting, or e-mailing your boyfriend. Also, stay away from the computer altogether so that you aren't tempted to check his Facebook status. Remember that you've got enough pain to deal with right now; there's no need to add to it. Are you on board with this?"

If the client commits to putting the plan into action, the next step usually is to troubleshoot potential barriers. In contrast with individual therapy sessions, where the clinician might give the client more time to come up with such barriers on her or his own, the clinician generally will take a more active and directive role in phone coaching. The clinician might simply ask the client if specific barriers are relevant, as seen in the example below:

THERAPIST: Let's talk about stuff that might get in the way of this plan. Based on past calls, I wonder if you might forget or decide you don't want to do it.

CLIENT: I really don't think that's going to happen this time. I know I'm not going to solve this problem overnight. I know the best thing for me is to just ride it out until we can meet.

THERAPIST: I'm really glad to hear that, and I totally agree. What if, by chance, you end up seeing another reminder of your boyfriend, checking his Facebook page, etc.?

CLIENT: I know I'm going to be tempted, but I know it's not a good idea.

THERAPIST: OK, so can we agree that, if you do slip up, you will go right back to your plan? Get yourself back to the schedule for distracting and soothing activities, and if you can't do anything else, just get yourself to bed. Also, remember the skills for dealing with self-harm urges. I'm thinking you should probably take those out of your binder and put them someplace where you can see them.

CLIENT: OK, I'll do that right now. I might need them.

THERAPIST: Is there anything that we're missing here? Anything that could possibly get in the way of our plan that we haven't discussed yet?

On the other hand, if the client seems reluctant to try the plan, the clinician might use strategies to help the client commit to the plan. Again, it is important to remember that time is short, and the clinician does not have much time to enhance the client's motivation or commitment. In individual DBT or CBT sessions, the clinician might use several different motivational or commitment strategies to help the client commit to change (see Linehan, 1993a; see also Miller & Rollnick, 2013). On the phone, the clinician should be prepared to use similar strategies in an abbreviated way. Clinicians might be tempted to go to great lengths to "convince" the client to implement the plan, particularly when the client has called reporting urges to engage in self-injury or suicidal behavior. In these cases, the clinician must balance the risk of self-injury or suicidal behavior with the risk of reinforcing noncompliance by providing increased time and attention when the client is unwilling to try skills. This topic will be discussed further in Chapter 7 (focused on suicide crisis calls).

Applying the 24-Hour Rule

At times, the clinician discovers that the client has self-injured or attempted suicide less than 24 hours before the call. I do not routinely ask at the beginning of calls whether my clients have done anything to harm themselves, but this is certainly one way to find out. In my experience, clients often spontaneously report this either during the call or in a voice message prior to the call, and the topic also often comes up when I ask what coping methods the client has already tried. At other times, however, the clinician might not know until the next therapy session. In that case, the clinician should try to ensure that the client informs her about self-injury or suicidal behavior at the beginning of any subsequent calls.

When the 24-hour rule is in effect, the goals and structure of a phone coaching call are different from what I have described above. The primary goals for these calls are to ensure safety and reduce the chances of serious physical harm or death, and to avoid inadvertently reinforcing self-injury or suicidal behavior. The structure of the calls is geared toward these goals, and the calls are even briefer than standard phone coaching calls.

The clinician generally starts off by reminding the client of the rule, briefly assessing whether medical attention is required, or the client is at imminent suicide risk. If there is a reason to suspect the need for medical intervention, the clinician helps the client access medical help. Since many clinicians conducting phone coaching are not medical practitioners, I suggest that clinicians recommend and attempt to facilitate medical intervention if there is any indication that it might be needed. Some indications could include evidence of severe loss of blood, wounds that might require stitches, signs of infection (e.g., fever, hardening around the tissue, visible signs such as redness), grogginess, nausea, slurred speech, incoherence, and so forth. It can be helpful to have a medical colleague to consult with about these circumstances. If there is evidence of ongoing imminent suicide risk, the clinician should follow some of the steps outlined in Chapter 7, pertaining to the management of suicide risk during suicide crisis calls. In either of these situations, I recommend that the clinician take a matter-of-fact approach, avoid providing more support or validation than the client normally receives when she has not harmed herself, and consult and debrief with a colleague soon after the phone call.

When the clinician does not need to take steps to ensure medical safety or reduce ongoing suicide risk, she should end the call as quickly as possible. Clients experience a variety of negative reactions in this scenario, including embarrassment, shame, hurt feelings, sadness, anger (toward self or clinician), or frustration; thus, the clinician should end the call compassionately, with consideration of how difficult this situation might be for the client (i.e., avoid saying or inadvertently conveying, "Sucks to be you!"). It can also be difficult for the clinician to end the call. I have only had to do this a handful of times, but I've often felt guilty, concerned that I've rejected or hurt the client's feelings, and worried about the client's well-being. Sometimes, effective therapy requires the therapist to make emotionally challenging decisions. It can help, therefore, to have a support system of colleagues who can buttress the clinician's use of the 24-hour rule and reaffirm that the decision to get off the phone was reasonable. The example below illustrates the scenario in which a therapist ends a call after finding out that the client had cut himself less than 24 hours ago:

CLIENT: I had a really hard time waiting for your call.

THERAPIST: I'm sorry it took so long for me to get back to you. I was busy in back-to-back appointments for much of the day. Did you manage to use your skills and avoid hurting yourself?

CLIENT: Ummm . . .

THERAPIST: Yes?

CLIENT: Well, I actually ended up cutting myself. Why is this so important, like the first thing you're asking me?

THERAPIST: Hey, I think you know why it's important. We've talked about this more than a few times before. When did you cut yourself?

CLIENT: Around 2:00 P.M. or so. It was pretty minor, and I stopped before I got too far.

THERAPIST: I'm glad to hear that, and I'm still sorry to hear you ended up cutting yourself. You know that means we can't talk, right? You remember the 24-hour rule?

CLIENT: I know, that's what I was afraid of. I still need help, though. Can't we just make an exception. I tried really hard for so many hours!

THERAPIST: I'm torn because I have no doubt you really tried hard. At the same time, I think we have to be really careful about this. I don't want there to be any chance that my talking to you will increase your risk in the future. So, I'm going to have to be firm about the rule. Let me check, though. You said the cutting was minor. Do you have any reason to think you might need stitches or medical attention?

CLIENT: No, it's not even deep or anything. I cleaned and disinfected it, and I used gauze and stuff.

THERAPIST: OK, good. Are you having any suicide urges, thoughts, or plans?

CLIENT: No, I sort of was before, but not since I cut myself.

THERAPIST: All right, so we're going to have to finish up now, and I'll look forward to seeing you in a couple of days on Tuesday . . .

The above example illustrates how brief phone coaching calls can be when the 24-hour rule is in effect. One concern is that the clinician ends the call when the client says she's not suicidal but may need to remain on the phone a little longer if she is suicidal. The risk is that additional attention and help might reinforce suicidality. To minimize this risk, the clinician should engage in very brief, pointed risk assessment and err on the side of caution. If the client does not quickly commit to follow a safety or crisis plan, remove lethal means, or take further steps (as needed) to reduce risk, the clinician might need to have the client go to the hospital, contact loved ones, call 911, or engage in other actions to reduce risk. Strategies for suicide crisis calls are further discussed in Chapter 7 and can be helpful in this situation. I recommend that the clinician take approaches that are more conservative and less desirable to the client in order to avoid reinforcing suicidality.

There are a couple of other important considerations regarding the 24-hour rule. First, the clinician should avoid the temptation to reassure the client by stating that a call will be forthcoming after the 24-hour period is up. Some students and clinicians learning DBT fall into the trap of scheduling or encouraging a call as soon as the 24 hours has lapsed. This could easily set up a reinforcing system whereby the client self-injures or attempts suicide and then automatically has contingent communication with the clinician after 24 hours. Second, the clinician should always debrief phone coaching calls in the next therapy session, particularly if they have enacted 24-hour rule that week.

Debriefing Phone Coaching in Individual Therapy Sessions

Clinicians should regularly debrief with the client regarding phone coaching calls that have occurred since the last session. Such debriefing discussions are much like the postgame debriefing that commonly occurs after professional sports game broadcasts. Following a challenging game, broadcasters review the coach's feedback, what the team did well, areas for improvement, and plans for future games. Similarly, debriefing phone coaching can help solidify the skills the client used to effectively navigate a difficult situation and facilitate planning for similar situations. Reflecting on effective (or ineffective) skill use can help the client remember what to do or avoid in future situations. Debriefing also can address ways to generalize skills the client found helpful to other situations. To help shape the client's autonomy with skills (and facilitate generalization beyond the end of therapy), there might be a plan for the client to use skills that worked following this or previous calls before calling the clinician the next time.

Debriefing also can help the clinician and client to proactively address or prevent problems with phone coaching. Setting a norm of debriefing phone coaching can help to prevent problems and therapy-interfering behaviors (TIBs) from persisting. I have noticed that many phone coaching challenges arise partly because the clinician has not brought these problems to the client's attention. The client regularly calls too frequently, for too long, or is hostile on the phone (or via electronic communication). The clinician has begun to dread the client's calls, but she or he still doesn't address these problems until several weeks have passed. By that point, the clinician is headed for burnout and is not in top shape emotionally to navigate the conversation. Furthermore, the client is confused as to why the clinician is only now raising concerns. The conversation goes poorly, and the clinician is even more reluctant in the future to bring up problems with phone coaching. A consistent routine of talking about phone coaching every session can prevent this problematic cycle, catching problems before they balloon and become difficult to manage. When debriefing addresses phone coaching-related TIB, it can be helpful to use some of the strategies I discuss in Chapter 8.

There is no set structure for debriefing phone coaching. One of the requirements of an adherent individual DBT session is for the therapist to check on and discuss other modes of treatment, such as skills training and phone coaching, at some point during the therapy session. Whether the treatment is DBT, CBT, or some other approach, making this kind of debriefing a routine component of each therapy session allows ample time to address problems or concerns and minimizes the chance that the clinician will forget to discuss phone coaching. I generally try to do this toward the beginning of every therapy session after we have set the session agenda, mainly so I don't forget to do it later on. Some helpful debriefing questions are presented below.

- "How did you feel about our phone call on Thursday?"
- "What was most helpful about our calls this week?"
- "What can we do to make phone coaching more effective for you?"
- "Which skills worked best?"
- "Which skills do you think you need more practice with?"
- "What's your plan for practicing these skills?"
- "Did you learn anything new that you can use in similar situations?"
- "What's your plan for this week?"
- "What about the next time a similar situation comes up?"

When debriefing addresses TIB, it can be helpful to put TIB on the agenda for the session and carve out an appropriate amount of time to discuss it. The clinician might briefly highlight and put concerns about phone coaching on the agenda. A clinician might say, for example, "I'd like to spend some time today talking about how phone coaching went this week. I'm really glad I was able to help you. I also noticed that we spoke several times, and our calls were a little longer than I'd like them to be. I'd like us to discuss ways to make sure phone coaching keeps working well for both of us. What are your thoughts?" As discussions of TIB around phone coaching can sometimes be emotionally evocative, I do not recommend that clinicians dive in and have these discussions at the very beginning of the therapy session, before the game plan (agenda) for the session is clear. Challenging discussions of phone coaching may last well beyond the agenda-setting portion of the session, leaving little time to organize goals or agenda items and address other important topics.

Being Dialectical about Structure

The key dialectical tension when it comes to structuring is that of rigidity versus flexibility. This is much like the dialectic of a protocol- versus principle-driven treatment. DBT has protocols and is principle-driven (Linehan, 1993a). Similarly, when it comes to phone coaching, rigidity and structure have value, for many of the reasons discussed in this chapter. A clear routine and structure can help the client feel anchored, regulated, and organized when she is caught in the storm of her emotions. Structure can help the client and clinician accomplish skills coaching in an efficient, helpful manner. Flexibility, however, also has value. What if the client calls because a family member has just passed away and just needs to talk for the first several minutes? What if the client calls in the middle of your meal in a restaurant, seeking skills to avoid going on a bender? Or, the client calls as he is walking toward a bridge he plans to jump off? What if all the client needs is a few quick words of encouragement to use skills she already knows how to use, to get out of bed in the morning, or to make it to today's session? What if the client is calling to report progress? In many of these situations, it would be peculiar and ineffective to stick rigidly to the structure and guidelines described above, although the general principles (targeting, effectively managing contingencies, etc.) often still apply. One synthesis of this dialectic of rigidity versus flexibility is for the clinician to have these practical recommendations and guidelines burned into her brain, but remain willing to go "off-script" so to speak, always keeping core DBT principles in mind. As recommended in Chapter 2, the clinician also should have some kind of network of colleagues to consult with and ensure that she is acting ineffectively by going off the script or sticking too closely to the script.

Summary

In summary, structuring phone coaching calls can help the clinician and the client maximize their use of time on the phone. The clinician should organize time according to the DBT hierarchy of phone coaching targets, which includes (in order) reducing life-threatening behavior, increasing skills generalization, and decreasing a sense of conflict or alienation from the clinician. It also is important to effectively manage contingencies during phone coaching by reinforcing effective behavior and avoiding the reinforcement of ineffective behavior. During the beginning of the call, the clinician typically briefly orients the client to the focus of the call, placing emphasis on skills coaching; briefly assesses the problem prompting the call; and emphasizes the norm/expectation that the client has already tried skills before calling the clinician. During the middle section of the call, the clinician's primary aim is to provide effective skills coaching. To facilitate skills coaching, the clinician will find it helpful to direct the flow of the conversation and to use contingency management strategies to differentially reinforce effective behavior. When wrapping up the call, one key aim is to help the client commit to a plan involving skills and troubleshoot barriers to this plan. When a client calls less than 24 hours after life-threatening behavior, the clinician's primary aims are to ensure safety and avoid inadvertently reinforcing the life-threatening behavior. As such, the clinician usually briefly reminds the client of the 24-hour rule, assesses whether the client is medically safe, and promptly ends the call. The clinician also may need to assess and intervene regarding suicide risk, using some of the strategies discussed in Chapter 7. It is also helpful for the clinician to regularly debrief phone coaching during the next individual therapy session. Overall, when the clinician appropriately and consistently structures phone coaching calls, phone coaching generally goes smoothly and helps clients learn to put their skills into action in her or his everyday life. Finally, one important dialectic to keep in mind regarding the structuring of phone coaching is that of rigidity versus flexibility.

CHAPTER 5

Core DBT Skills Coaching Principles and Strategies

G iven the emphasis in phone coaching on skills coaching as a means to generalize new behaviors, the clinician should be aware of key coaching principles and strategies. Some of these principles are specific to DBT, but all are grounded in behavioral theory and evidence-based practices. This chapter begins with a discussion of ways to tailor skills training and coaching to a client's capabilities. Effective skills coaching requires some awareness of the client's position on the learning curve for certain skills. Subsequently, I discuss key principles and strategies used to coach clients in skills, emphasizing keen observation (and mindfulness) on the part of the clinician, the prompting of new behavior, and the effective use of instruction and feedback. Many of the principles and strategies discussed in this chapter also are applicable to coaching occurring in the context of other modes of treatment, such as in individual or group therapy, or treatment occurring in milieu settings, where phone coaching often is not feasible. Although I emphasize phone coaching, my aim is for this chapter to be useful for clinicians coaching skills in a variety of contexts, including individual treatment, milieu or residential settings, and group treatment.

Tailoring Skills Training and Coaching to a Client's Capabilities

To effectively coach clients on skill use, you need to determine how far along the learning curve the client is with respect to certain skills. Some clients already have learned the skills they need to get through a tough situation, whereas, for others, the skills they need feel like a foreign language. As the clinician's skills teaching and coaching strategies should differ in these two situations, knowing what level a client is at can help the clinician to use coaching strategies that best fit the needs of the client. In DBT, we find it useful to consider three different levels of skill attainment or learning: skill acquisition, strengthening, and generalization (for a more extensive discussion of this topic, please see Farmer & Chapman, 2016; Linehan, 2015). Within this section, I discuss these three stages and their implications for both skills training and coaching, as training and coaching often go hand-in-hand, and coaching is most effective when the clinician knows how to teach skills.

In the *acquisition phase,* the client is first learning a new skill or behavior. She may have very little knowledge of or experience with the skill. This situation is akin to a client who needs coaching in distress tolerance skills but hasn't gotten to that module in a DBT skills training group, or a client who needs coaching on anxiety management (e.g., diaphragmatic breathing) but hasn't learned any anxiety management skills. Skills training in the acquisition phase has the key goals of helping the client (1) become inspired and motivated to use the skill, (2) learn what the skill entails, (3) understand when and why to use it, and (4) get her feet wet with the skill. Key skills training strategies include specifically describing and operationalizing the skill, explaining the rationale for the skill, explaining when and why to use it, modeling or demonstrating the skill (or making use of peer or other models or examples of the use of the skill), and encouraging the client to get her feet wet by trying it out.

Skills coaching has similar goals. If I'm coaching a client in how to use diaphragmatic breathing, I want to inspire the client to try out the skill, explain how and why it works, and demonstrate it if possible by practicing it together or talking aloud while I practice it. The difference here is that, in skills training, there is plenty of time to teach the skill, whereas in phone coaching, I need to accomplish this quickly on the fly.

As an example, when I teach students a new way of kicking in martial arts, I might begin by describing exactly what the kick is supposed to look like, why it is effective, and when to use it. I also demonstrate what the kick looks like, describing the proper orientation of one's body, leg, and foot, and so on. I might also demonstrate or have an advanced student demonstrate the kick, and then have the students get a feel for the kick by trying it out a couple of times. At this acquisition stage, I'm not overly concerned whether the students are performing the kick perfectly (provided that they are not doing it in a way that will cause injury); I'm more concerned that they understand the principles behind it and that they start to get a feel for it. I also want to energize and inspire them to use it. It's not easy to learn new, complicated techniques, and it helps when the instructor is able to get the students excited about doing so.

When coaching during the acquisition phase, I use shaping principles and begin by providing positive feedback when the students try to perform the kick. As mentioned, I want to encourage students to try it out and provide immediate reinforcement (or at least, what I hope will be reinforcement) when they do. I emphasize positive feedback on what the students are doing properly more so than feedback on what to change or adjust. This is because it can also be overwhelming and confusing to receive a lot of corrective feedback when a skill is completely new. I also encourage the student to use the kick in easy practice scenarios, rather than to try it out while sparring with an advanced student.

Similarly, to help a client understand a psychosocial skill and why it might help, the clinician provides clear instructions on the skill along with a rationale for why it might be helpful for the client's specific situation. To encourage the client to try out and "play" with the skill, the clinician also inspires and encourages the client to use the skill, and where possible, emphasizes positive feedback on what the client is doing effectively. The clinician tries to reinforce efforts to use the skill and encourages the client to try the new skill in situations that are not particularly difficult or stressful. This way, the client is likely to experience success with the skill and be more willing to try it in the future.

Many of these steps can occur in a more condensed manner in the context of phone coaching. If in talking with a client on the phone, and I think he would benefit from the skill of paced breathing (involving slow, diaphragmatic breathing that follows a specific pattern, ideally a longer inhale than exhale; Linehan, 2015), I might approach coaching in the manner shown in the example below.

THERAPIST: OK, so from what you've told me, your anxiety and agitation are through the roof, and you're having a hard time thinking of what to do.

CLIENT: That's right, I can't . . . I just don't know what to do. I can't do that stuff we talked about. I don't even remember it.

THERAPIST: That's fine, that's what it's like when emotions are extremely high. You sort of reach your breakdown point and can't think. So, our goal is to get your emotions to the point where you can think. Sound OK?

CLIENT: Yeah.

THERAPIST: Here's a skill that will really help. It's called paced breathing. Paced breathing slows down your breathing, helps you get enough oxygen but not too much, and most importantly, slows your heart rate.

CLIENT: OK

THERAPIST: I think this is really going to help you. It's something you can do almost anywhere, and for some people, it has a pretty fast calming effect. It helps me a lot when I'm anxious about giving a talk or attending a stressful meeting, or when I'm really worried or angry. I know we haven't covered this in group yet, but are you willing to try it?

CLIENT: Yeah, I can try.

THERAPIST: OK, first, put one hand on your chest and the other on your abdomen. I'll do the same. Got that?

CLIENT: Yep.

THERAPIST: Now, focus on drawing air in through your abdomen and not your chest. Chest breathing can just make you more anxious.

CLIENT: I think I've heard of this before, and it didn't work.

THERAPIST: That's probably because you did the abdomen part but not the other more important part. The more important part is to breathe in for less time than you breathe out. OK, so follow me. I'm going to say, "In, 2, 3." When I do that, breathe in until I finish saying "3." Got it?

CLIENT: So far.

THERAPIST: Then, I'm going to say, "Out, 2, 3, 4, 5, 6." Exhale until I finish saying "6." OK, let's try it. If you feel lightheaded or can't breathe out for that long, let me know.

In this example, the therapist quickly provides the rationale for paced breathing, emphasizing how this skill will help and hopefully inspire the client to use it, provides brief instructions, and then quickly initiates a guided practice. The goal here is not for the client to master the skill, but rather to help him try it and see if it helps. In the future, he can practice regularly (to strengthen the skill) and try paced breathing in a variety of situations (to generalize the skill to other situations). It may be difficult at first to try a new skill in the situation above, but starting on the phone with the therapist likely would be easier than starting alone. If the client, with the therapist's help, finds the skill helpful, he may be willing to continue to use it when he gets off the phone.

A second important phase involves *skill strengthening*. Clients are in the skill-strengthening phase when they have demonstrated that they understand and can perform the skill correctly. At this point, the clinician facilitates regular practice and provides feedback to help the client hone and refine the skill (Farmer & Chapman, 2016). The clinician might assign relevant homework assignments, prompt the client to practice the skill during sessions, provide feedback, and coach the client in effective skill use. Compared with the skill acquisition phase, there is less emphasis on instruction or helping the client understand the skill. Rather, the emphasis is on helping the client to effectively perform the skill. Once a student can perform a martial arts kick appropriately, for example, I set up different practice scenarios requiring the student to engage in high-frequency practice (to make the movements more automatic); maintain proper body, leg, and foot positioning (to refine the movements); and to deploy the kick as quickly as possible (to make the new kick more automatic or instinctual). Subsequently, I encourage the student to use the kick in increasingly challenging situations (e.g., sparring). Similarly, I might encourage a client learning the interpersonal effectiveness skill of *validation* (part of the "GIVE" skills in DBT; Linehan, 1993b, 2015) to practice validation during practice drills in skills training sessions as well as in everyday life. Practice exercises might focus on increasingly difficult situations, such as conflict, disagreements, and so forth.

With these basic principles in mind, the clinician can approach phone coaching with the aim of strengthening the client's skills. Let's say that the client above understands and has learned paced breathing and other skills to reduce emotional arousal. This time, he is calling for help with intense anger.

THERAPIST: How about you briefly summarize what's happening.

CLIENT: I just don't know what to do, I'm so enraged with my sister. She keeps telling me I should be doing more to support our mother [who recently was in a car accident]. I already feel guilty enough about it. She just doesn't get what it's like to have such a hard time even getting out of bed. Why would she want to make it worse! I just want to tell her I'm done with her.

THERAPIST: It seems unfair that your sister is criticizing you when you're doing your best to keep your head above water. I know well that you already feel guilty enough!

CLIENT: Yeah, that's true.

THERAPIST: I can see how you'd be angry. How high is your anger right now?

CLIENT: I don't know, through the roof! Maybe 9 or 10. I should just call her now and tell her to fuck off for good. It's about time. Maybe you could help me do that.

THERAPIST: Do you think now is the best time to call your sister?

CLIENT: I don't know, I guess not.

THERAPIST: Probably not, no point in making things worse. I know that happened last time. Things blew up, and you ended up really distraught. It's hard, though, because you're stuck with all of this anger. Would you say you're at your skill breakdown point [the point where it's hard to think clearly or use complicated skills]?

CLIENT: Yeah, probably.

THERAPIST: Are you willing to get your anger down a bit so we can think about what to do next?

CLIENT: I guess I can try.

THERAPIST: OK, good, let's table the idea of talking with your sister for now. Let's practice paced breathing instead. We've done this before, so go ahead and try it on the phone with me for 2 minutes. Hold the phone close so I can hear how it's going. I'll tell you when the time's up.

CLIENT: All right.

THERAPIST: Time's not up yet, but good job with slow breathing. I can hear that your exhale is about the same as your inhale. Try to make the exhale longer. Remember, exhaling reduces your heart rate. Maybe blow the air out like you're blowing through a large straw or something.

CLIENT: Oh, right. OK.

THERAPIST: OK, time's up. How high is your anger right now?

CLIENT: I guess I feel a little calmer, and my muscles feel kind of relaxed. Maybe 5 or 6. I still feel pretty bitter.

THERAPIST: Paced breathing can work pretty well for anger, and I can see why you'd feel bitter. Do you think the anger is down enough so you can think clearly about what to do next?

CLIENT: Yeah, I don't know. I think I should just leave it for this evening. Nothing's going to change anyway.

THERAPIST: That sounds like wise thinking to me. Maybe we could talk about how to deal with your sister next time we meet.

CLIENT: That's a good plan. Thanks. If I don't bring it up with her eventually, I'll just keep simmering. I mean, this just keeps happening.

THERAPIST: I know. I agree. I think you guys should have a heart-to-heart talk, using your interpersonal effectiveness skills, but not when you're through-the-roof angry. Here's what I'd like you to try: When we get off the phone, try the paced breathing for about 10 minutes, and check whether you've been able to get closer to wise mind. Then, write out a little script of what you would like to say to your sister. I think this will help you express yourself, and this can help you stop ruminating. I often find that myself. If I write stuff out in a skillful way, not just venting, I don't ruminate as much. Plus, it's good practice with your interpersonal skills. Then, just leave it, and we can look at it together on Thursday and maybe do some practicing. Hold off on talking with her until after that. Sound OK?

In this example, as the client already has learned paced breathing, the therapist doesn't spend time describing the skill or providing the rationale for it. Instead, she prompts the client to try it. She provides positive feedback, but noticing that the skill likely would be more effective if he were to extend his exhalations, she makes a suggestion on how to do this. The aim is to help the client more effectively use the skill. She also takes a more advanced approach than in the original scenario, asking the client to combine paced breathing with other skills he has learned, specifically using interpersonal effectiveness skills to come up with a script of what to say to his sister. Because of the limited time available in phone coaching, she suggests that he bring this script to the next session so they can refine and practice it before he speaks with his sister.

A third phase, after the client has acquired and made inroads in strengthening a skill, involves *skill generalization,* as shown by the effective use of skills in a variety of situations. A client who successfully uses interpersonal effectiveness skills with the therapist but falters with others (partner, coworkers, etc.) has not successfully generalized these skills. Often, to generalize skills, the client must practice them in diverse situations, not just in the therapy room. The clinician's job, therefore, is to help the client identify relevant situations and encourage her to practice skills in these situations. Phone coaching is a vehicle for the clinician to help the client apply skills in diverse and highly stressful situations. The hope is that, over time, the clinician's guidance and coaching will help the client benefit from skills wherever they are needed.

Several methods can encourage generalization during phone coaching. If a client, for example, has effectively used interpersonal effectiveness skills in nondemanding situations, the clinician might encourage the practice of interpersonal skills in more challenging contexts, such as interpersonal conflict. A client who has primarily used opposite action to approach feared situations might be encouraged to try it out when the predominant emotion is anger rather than fear (see Chapman & Gratz, 2015, for applications of various DBT skills to anger). The clinician might also encourage generalization by explicitly relating situations occurring during phone coaching to situations in the client's daily life. If the client, for example, is frustrated with the clinician and feels invalidated or unsupported on the phone, it might be effective to relate this experience to other relationships (either during phone coaching or during the next therapy session). I have often found that the interpersonal problems my clients experience in other relationships regularly show up during phone coaching calls. This can make phone coaching challenging, but presents opportunities to help the client deal with pervasive difficulties that hamper other relationships.

While debriefing phone coaching from the previous week, the clinician might relate situations discussed during phone coaching to other situations in the client's life. We were seeing a client who called for phone coaching after becoming suicidal following the tragedy in Charlottesville, Virginia. She is a transgendered woman, and she was afraid that she would be victimized and worried that she would continue to be saddled with the burden of fighting injustice for the rest of her life. While debriefing the phone coaching call, the clinician had the opportunity to further assess factors contributing to the client's suicidality. It turned out that, when the client experiences reminders of discrimination against trans-gendered individuals or other minorities (either through direct discrimination or news stories, conversations with friends, etc.), she often feels a general sense of lack of safety and uncertainty about her safety as well as sadness that she can't be who she is without being at higher risk than others. These experiences spiral into hopeless thoughts and sometimes suicidal thoughts and urges. After illuminating this important broader pattern, the clinician and client worked on skills to address it, primarily including the DBT skills of radical acceptance and problem solving (taking steps to get involved in advocacy work).

Key Component of Skills Coaching

The primary aim of skills coaching is to help the client effectively apply skills in relevant situations. The clinician can use a variety of strategies to accomplish this goal during phone coaching or other forms of coaching, such as coaching in milieu settings. In this section, I discuss several of these strategies, including (1) assessing the situation; (2) instructing (including verbally instructing the client, modeling, or demonstrating the skill as needed) the client in the use of a skill; (3) prompting the client to use the skill(s); (4) observing the client's behavior; (5) providing feedback; (6) prompting the client to use the skill again, incorporating the clinician's feedback; and (7) repeating this process as needed.

Assessing the Situation

The key step of assessing the situation prompting a phone coaching call already was discussed in Chapter 4; thus, the focus here is on assessment in settings where the clinician is using milieu coaching or coaching in an individual therapy session. I have worked and consulted in various residential or correctional treatment settings and have found that a good start in assessing the situation is to observe client behavior. I was working at a residential facility for residents with developmental disabilities who had committed sexual offenses, and one of the residents often became agitated and aggressive very quickly when provoked by another resident. The early signs of agitation usually involved fidgeting, pacing quickly and aimlessly, and clearing his throat. When I observed these signs, I would try to casually walk up to him in a nonthreatening manner and assess the situation. I'd ask him what was up, and he'd often tell me something another resident did that bothered him (taking his things, changing the TV channel, teasing him, etc.). Although he was not adept at describing how he felt, it was often clear that he was agitated and frustrated. I briefly coached him on skills he could use, primarily gentle avoidance and distraction, and watched him do it. Until he seemed much calmer, I stayed close by so I could give him further coaching as needed and ideally prevent him from ditching the skills and attacking the other resident.

In an individual therapy session, the therapist may similarly use observation to determine whether a client needs in-the-moment coaching on a skill. The client may, for example, be sobbing unremittingly, appear agitated or like he is experiencing very strong emotions, engaging in angry or threatening behavior, demonstrating a discrepancy between what he is saying (e.g., talking about a devastating recent breakup) and how he is saying it (talking about this breakup in a cavalier manner), seem to be avoiding particular emotions or topics, and so forth. In DBT, the most common cue suggesting the need for in-the-moment coaching is evidence that a client is emotionally dysregulated. When a therapist observes this, she might assess the client's current experience, try to determine what prompting event(s) seem to have cued or preceded the emotion dysregulation, determine whether a skill might help the client regulate his emotions, suggest this skill, and take some of the other steps described below.

Instructing on Skill Use

Once the situation or problem requiring skills coaching is clear, a helpful next step is to instruct the client on how to use a relevant skill or set of skills. For clients who are just learning a new skill (skill acquisition phase), the therapist might spend time describing the skill, clarifying what it is and when and how to use it, and be sure the client has a clear rationale for using the skill. Clients who are further along in the learning process (skill strengthening) might simply need to be reminded of the skill and how to apply it to the current situation (skill generalization).

At times, clients already are using potentially effective skills but need help with them. In this case, the clinician might help the client figure out how to make the skill work better, or whether it needs to be used differently in a particular situation. A client might, for example, say that she has been trying to use the mindfulness skill of observing, but is "failing" because she is ruminating or having many worry thoughts. In this case, the clinician might remind the client that mindful observing does not require a blank mind devoid of thoughts. Rather, the practice of observing involves the client gently guiding her mind back to her experience of the present moment whenever she drifts onto the thought train. Thus, the client should focus on gently guiding her mind to the present whenever it wanders. Sometimes, this type of instruction or clarification is enough for the client to move forward and use the skill effectively. The example below begins after the clinician has used the standard structural strategies for the beginning segment of the call (described in Chapter 3).

THERAPIST: OK, so you're having difficulty coping with anxiety about the job interview for tomorrow, and you're trying to be mindful of your emotions, is that right?

CLIENT: Yeah, but it's so hard! I think I'm doing it wrong. The anxiety keeps coming back, and my thoughts are driving me crazy. I just keep thinking about what if I totally screw up or say something bizarre. I'm really scared. I mean, if I don't get a job soon, I won't even be able to afford therapy.

THERAPIST: I know this interview is bringing up a ton of anxiety for you, and it can be hard to ride it out while you wait for tomorrow. It's great to hear that you're trying mindfulness. That skill could really help you get through this. Sounds like the main problem is that you're getting stuck on worry thoughts, and this makes you think you're doing something wrong.

CLIENT: Yeah, I can't even focus on my anxiety without all of these stupid thoughts stirring everything back up again.

THERAPIST: Well, that's not surprising; it's hard to focus when you're feeling really anxious. Remember that mindfulness won't get rid of your thoughts, but it will help you let them go. I also think it will help you learn how to tolerate your anxiety without acting on it, like without cancelling the interview. Do you have urges to do that, by any chance?

CLIENT: Of course, just like last time. I'm really tempted to just e-mail and say I'm sick or not interested anymore.

THERAPIST: Remember what I always say: Avoid avoiding! I'm confident that you can get through this interview. We've done a lot of practice. You did really well, even when I asked you tough questions. For mindfulness of current emotions, remember that it's OK to have thoughts. Thoughts are totally normal. Your brain is naturally going to come up with a lot of worry thoughts when you're anxious. Don't try to get rid of them. Just tell yourself, "another worry thought," and focus on the sensations of your anxiety. I wouldn't suggest that you do this all night, though. So, I'd suggest you try it for about 15–30 minutes, and then use some of your self-soothing or relaxation skills. How does that sound?

CLIENT: OK, I'll try that.

THERAPIST: OK, great. One more thing: It can also be helpful to sit in a relaxed, open position when you're trying to be mindful of sensations of anxiety. Try doing the "willing hands" posture we covered in group last week, where your hands are open on your lap. [To be continued below.]

In this example, beyond validating, encouraging the client to avoid avoiding, and making hopeful statements about the job interview, the clinician primarily used the strategy of instructing the client on skill use. She normalized the client's experience of worry thoughts, provided some instructions on how to make the skill of mindfulness of current emotions more effective (label worry thoughts, use the skill for about 30 minutes before moving on to other skills), and instructed the client on which other skills to try (distraction and self-soothing). Given enough time, the clinician might also take the next step and prompt the client to practice the skill while she is on the phone.

Prompting Skill Practice

Prompting skill practice involves having the client practice a skill, ideally on the phone (or in the milieu or individual/group therapy session) with the clinician. In DBT, this is also often called *dragging out new behavior*. Compared with simply instructing a client to try out a skill on her or his own, prompting skill practice has a few key advantages. First, the client has the opportunity to gain further practice and experience how the skill might work, with the clinician available for any questions that might arise. If the client simply tries a skill independently, the opportunities to ask questions, receive guidance, or clear up any confusion about the skill are limited. This situation is akin to a piano teacher simply providing verbal instructions on how to play a song without having the student try it out before going home to practice. A second advantage is that observations of how the client is using the skill can provide useful assessment information, generating hypotheses about areas of strength and behavioral deficits to work on in therapy. A third related advantage is that, with this information, the clinician will be able to provide immediate coaching and feedback. Clients are likely to learn more from feedback occurring close in time to their use of a skill compared to feedback occurring a week later in the therapy session.

One challenge for the prompting of skill practice during skills coaching is that it is much easier to find the time to prompt clients to use skills in prolonged therapy sessions than it is during a brief call, or a brief coaching session in the milieu. The clinician should, therefore, prompt skill use quickly and efficiently. The clinician must quickly recognize and jump on opportunities to ask the client to try out a skill. To illustrate how the clinician might do this, I have continued the example above regarding the client attempting to use mindfulness to ride out anxiety about a job interview:

THERAPIST: I want to see how this will work for you before we get off the phone. Let's take a minute and have you practice mindfulness of your current emotion in this new way, recognizing and labeling worry thoughts and coming back to your bodily sensations.

CLIENT: OK, I can give it a try, but I'm starting to feel panicky already.

THERAPIST: OK, so the first step is to slow down your breathing like we talked about before. Also, sit in a relaxed, open position with your hands open in your lap. Are you doing it?

CLIENT: Yes.

THERAPIST: Perfect, all right, now bring your attention to your body. Focus on the areas where you feel the anxiety. What are you noticing?

CLIENT: I feel most in my chest and my stomach. My stomach feels kind of sick, and my chest feels like there's a tight knot in it.

THERAPIST: OK, you're doing really well. Keep your attention focused on your stomach and your chest. Try to experience the sensations with some curiosity. See if they stay the same or change. Remember to label and let go of any worry thoughts. [To be continued below.]

Observing the Client's Practice of Skills

To be an excellent coach in any activity, whether it's sports, playing a musical instrument, or DBT skills, requires keen observation skills. The coach needs to be alert, attentive, and mindful of the student or client's behavior. I often help students prepare for their martial arts testing by having them practice the movements or sequences that they will soon be tested on. I've noticed that, after just an hour or two of this practice, I often want to lie down and take a nap. This is not because they're doing poorly but because, to provide good feedback, I need to concentrate on every detail of the students' movements. This kind of intense concentration can be exhausting. If my mind wanders and I don't bring it back quickly, I am likely to miss an error and an important opportunity to help the student perform a particular move correctly. And I certainly don't want to be the assistant instructor whose students end up doing poorly on the test!

During therapy sessions and phone coaching, it is similarly important for the clinician to mindfully observe the client's behavior. A clinician conducting exposure therapy, for example, must pay close attention to the client's verbal and nonverbal communication and attend to any signs that the client might be avoiding or dissociating (Abramowitz, 2013; Abramowitz, Deacon, & Whiteside, 2011; Craske, Treanor, Conway, Zbozinek, & Vervliet, 2014). A clinician helping a client practice an interpersonal skill must carefully observe the client's choice of words, voice tone, demeanor, and body language. This is relatively easy to do during milieu coaching or in person coaching in individual or group-therapy sessions. During phone coaching, however, the clinician's opportunity to observe the client's behavior is limited. To compensate for this limitation, it can be effective for clinicians to actively guide clients in their use of the skill and to ask the client to describe her or his experience during or after using the skill. The following continues from the example above:

THERAPIST: What are you noticing so far?

CLIENT: My stomach is feeling a little less sick, but the knot in my chest still feels pretty tight. It is changing a bit, though.

THERAPIST: That's a nice, specific description of your emotions. What are you doing now?

CLIENT: I'm thinking about blushing or stammering during the interview.

THERAPIST: OK, worry thoughts. Say out loud, "worry thoughts are coming up." Go ahead.

CLIENT: Worry thoughts are coming up.

THERAPIST: Now, direct your attention to your sensations again. Tell me what you're experiencing.

CLIENT: My muscles feel a little tense. My jaw is tight. I think I'm frustrated with this whole thing. It's so hard to stay focused with all of these annoying thoughts. I just can't seem to block them out.

THERAPIST: It's true, it's really frustrating. Remember, though, that you don't need to block anything out. In fact, the more you try to block out the worry thoughts, the harder this is going to be. As hard as it is, every time you have a worry thought, just say in your mind, "Another worry thought," and gently guide your attention back to your body. Keep this up, and I think you'll find the thoughts a lot less maddening.

CLIENT: OK, I'll try to remember . . .

In this example, the clinician "observed" the client's skill practice by regularly asking him to describe what he was doing and experiencing. The client was using this skill effectively but needed some feedback about his attempts to block worry thoughts. In the next example, a client has called for help with stress-related to conflict with his roommate. He has been feeling angry and frustrated and experiencing urges to self-injure. In this call, the client and clinician have already discussed strategies to reduce the risk of self-injury. They also decided that interpersonal effectiveness skills would help the client communicate to the roommate that he needs some space and time alone this evening.

THERAPIST: OK, so go ahead and say it the way that you plan to say it to your roommate. Remember, describe the situation, express how you're feeling, ask for what you want, and let him know why it would be good for him to give you what you want. [These are the DEAR skills from DEAR MAN in the interpersonal effectiveness skills; see Linehan, 2014.]

CLINICIAN: OK . . . John, we've been arguing a lot over the last couple of days, and I'm feeling really stressed and frustrated. I just need you to get off my case this evening and leave me alone.

THERAPIST: OK, that's a really good start. I like the first part: you described the situation clearly and expressed how you were feeling using "I" statements. With a few tweaks, I think this would work even better. Although you asked for what you wanted, your voice tone came across as a little harsh. I'm also afraid that the words "get off my case" might just put your roommate on the defensive. Try saying, "I need some alone time this evening. Could we talk over coffee sometime tomorrow? My treat."

In this example, the clinician had the opportunity to observe and provide feedback on the client's phrasing and voice tone. In a therapy session, the clinician might have time to ask the client to assess her or his own skills. Indeed, improving self-observation and reflection can be one way to help facilitate the generalization of skills beyond therapy (as discussed in Chapter 9). During phone coaching, however, there may not be enough time to do this. As a result, it can be most effective to provide succinct and direct feedback.

Providing Feedback

Another important aspect of skills coaching involves the clinician providing the client with feedback on the use of particular skills. This feedback might be based on direct observations of the client using skills, the client's descriptions of attempts to use skills, information gleaned during debriefing following skills practice, or some combination of all three. Feedback based solely on a client's description of events, however, has limited benefits. A variety of factors may threaten the validity of client descriptions of past behavior, including common memory biases, impression management, and state-dependent recall, among others. Perhaps the most effective way to ensure that the clinician has accurate information is to directly observe the client using skills, as suggested above. This is one reason the strategy of prompting skill use or "dragging out new behavior" is so useful. Another helpful strategy is to encourage clients to use worksheets or take notes on their attempts to practice skills, and to have these notes available when they call the clinician for phone coaching. Feedback might address several different domains.

Feedback on the Client's Apparent Understanding of a Skill

The clinician might provide feedback on how well the client seems to understand the skill. Some clients have difficulty primarily because they have missed the main point of the skill. As in the example above, the client appeared to believe that mindfulness practice involves pushing away unwanted worry thoughts. I once saw a client who vehemently objected whenever we practiced mindfulness in our DBT skills group. She would say that mindfulness skills don't work and are completely useless. When I assessed what was troubling her about mindfulness skills, it became clear that she thought she needed to have a completely blank mind. She explained that she has attention-deficit/hyperactivity disorder (ADHD), and that her mind is always buzzing with thoughts. Mindfulness practice, of course, does not require a blank mind. Our minds are almost never devoid of thoughts. Indeed, some neuroscientists believe that the "default mode" for human cognitive activity involves a degree of daydreaming or flitting from one thought to another (Andrews-Hanna, 2011). When I explained this to the client, she breathed a sigh of relief and said that she would be willing to give mindfulness another try. Several weeks later, she came to group and reported that she had been finding her daily mindfulness practice to be very helpful in reducing stress and anxiety in her job as a primary school teacher.

Feedback on the Client's Performance of a Skill

Feedback might also focus on how the client is performing the skill. A tennis coach, for example, might give specific feedback on the student's stance or racket position, the angle of her or his swing during serving, and so forth. The goal is to help the client or student bring her or his behavior more closely in line with the skill.

As mentioned earlier, if a client is just learning the skill (skill acquisition phase), the clinician might emphasize positive feedback and deemphasize corrective feedback. To reinforce attempts to use the skill, the clinician might use praise or more natural forms of positive reinforcement whenever the client has even attempted a new skill. It also can be effective for the clinician to mindfully observe the client's behavior and pay close attention to what she or he is doing effectively. Validation of the client's experience and normalization of the difficulty of using a new skill in stressful circumstances can also be especially helpful.

The example the dialogue below involves a client who was trying to improve her sleep habits. Specifically, she was trying to establish a consistent rise time every morning (an important part of CBT for insomnia; Perlis, Jungquist, Smith, & Posner, 2006). She called because she was feeling increasingly stressed and agitated due to difficulties with insomnia. She was also feeling demoralized about her attempts to improve her sleep.

THERAPIST: How have things been going with the sleep schedule?

CLIENT: Not good.

THERAPIST: Oh, what hasn't been going well?

CLIENT: I just think I'm failing at this whole thing. I wasn't able to do it.

THERAPIST: That sounds really frustrating. Tell me what you did.

CLIENT: Well, I got up at 7:00 A.M. about two or three mornings over the last week.

THERAPIST: OK, and how many mornings do you normally wake up at the same time?

CLIENT: None, I guess. I mean, my sleep schedule is usually all over the place.

THERAPIST: OK, so if we're just looking at the 5-day workweek, it sounds like you've made about a 40–60% improvement over the past week. Does that sound about right?

CLIENT: Well, I guess when you put it that way . . .

THERAPIST: The thing is, changing your sleep schedule could be one of the hardest things you can do to take better care of yourself. A lot of people struggle to get themselves up at the same time every morning, even though they know this is a step toward overcoming insomnia. It seems to me that a 40–60% improvement in your first week is a lot of progress!

CLIENT: Thanks, I hadn't really thought of it that way. I just wish things were easier. I still sort of feel like I failed.

THERAPIST: You weren't by any chance thinking you would completely solve your insomnia this week? Or, maybe that it's sort of all or nothing?

CLIENT: OK, you got me. I know we've talked about that, but it still feels that way.

THERAPIST: Getting out of that thinking requires practice. Let's come back to that. For now, remember to pay attention to the small steps that you make. In fact, it might be better not to have a 100% success rate in your very first week. I think it's best to start small at a level that you can keep up for some time. So, I think you're right on track.

In this example, the clinician helped the client to view her progress in a different way. As this client is just learning better sleep habits, the clinician emphasized what the client was doing well rather than what the client was not doing well. The clinician also briefly targeted a problematic thinking pattern and provided some education on the importance of making small but sustainable changes in self-care practices.

Clients who are in the skill-strengthening phase, in contrast, often benefit from more specific corrective feedback to refine their use of a skill. In the example above, establishing a consistent sleep schedule was a completely new behavior. A continuation of this example is below. In this case, the same client already has learned the skills to manage anxiety and agitation, which also have been interfering with sleep.

THERAPIST: What have you been trying so far to cope with the anxiety and agitation?

CLIENT: I've been trying those TIPP skills [regulating strong emotional arousal by changing body temperature, engaging in intense exercise, or using paired relaxation or paced breathing strategies]. They work really well, but I just feel so wound up today. I put my face in cold water, and that helped for about 5 or 10 minutes. I've also been trying some of that paced breathing stuff.

THERAPIST: That's great, I think the TIP skills could really help. Tell me how you've been using paced breathing.

CLIENT: Just like we've been doing in skills group, I breathe in and count to 3, and I count to 6 while I'm breathing out. I'm just not noticing much of a difference, and I sort of feel like I'm not getting enough air.

THERAPIST: A lot of people feel that way for a while. It sounds like you're doing the counting properly. I have a guess about what might be going on. Try breathing in and out for about 20 seconds right now.

CLIENT: OK.

THERAPIST: What did you notice about your chest, abdomen, and shoulders when you breathed in and out?

CLIENT: I guess my shoulders were kind of moving up, and my chest was going in and out. My abdomen was moving a bit.

THERAPIST: Ah, I think that might be the problem. Remember how you're supposed to breathe through your abdomen or diaphragm?

CLIENT: Oh, right.

THERAPIST: You can tell you're not breathing through your diaphragm if your shoulders are rising whenever you breathe in, or if your chest is moving a lot. Let's try this together for about 30 seconds. Do the counting like you were doing it before, but try to make the hand on your abdomen move more than the hand on your chest.

CLIENT: You know, I really hate doing that because it just reminds me of how much weight I've gained.

THERAPIST: I know, I remember that. This might be a good opportunity to practice letting go of thoughts about your weight. And, once were done, if you're getting the hang of it, you don't have to put your hand on your abdomen anymore. Are you willing to give it a try?

CLIENT: OK.

THERAPIST: What's your level of anxiety right now?

CLIENT: I'd say around 60 or 65. It helps a bit to be talking with you.

THERAPIST: I'm glad to hear that. OK, now let's give the breathing a try for a minute or so . . . How was it? What's your anxiety like now?

CLIENT: That was better. I mean, I'm still at around 50, but it's taking the edge off.

THERAPIST: Great, and that was only after a minute or so. Try this out, remembering to breathe through your diaphragm, for about 5–10 minutes after we're finished talking, and see how it works.

In the example above, the therapist is focused on refinements that are needed for the skill to work better for the client. The therapist hypothesized that the client might have been engaging in chest breathing rather than diaphragmatic breathing, and she tested this hypothesis by having the client breathe and notice the movement in her chest and abdomen. After confirming the problem, the therapist provided feedback and prompted the client to practice again correctly. To get a rough gauge of how effective this adjustment was, the therapist also had the client rate her agitation before and after trying the skill.

Feedback on the Likely Effectiveness of the Client's Behavior

The clinician might also provide feedback and suggestions on the likely effectiveness of the client's use of a skill. In the previous example of the client struggling with conflict with a roommate, the clinician suggested that the client's use of the phrase "get off my case" could backfire. This type of feedback focusing on the likely effect of a behavior is also called *contingency clarification* in DBT (Linehan, 1993a). To effectively clarify contingencies, the clinician specifically describes the client's behavior and its likely consequences.

The clinician does not always know what these consequences might be, so in many cases the clinician simply makes reasonable hypotheses. These hypotheses ideally are related to the clinician's case formulation and knowledge of behavioral science and the skill the client is trying to use. We know, for example, that if a client is trying to learn to overcome fear of social situations but only engages in exposure with an object or person serving as a safety signal, the client is unlikely to learn that social situations are nonthreatening. Instead, the client may learn that social situations are nonthreatening as long as the safety signal is present (Blakey & Abramowitz, 2016; Dugas & Ladouceur, 2000). As another example, a clinician who is well informed about the research on self-regulation being a limited resource could clarify the likely consequences of the client's attempts to get through a stressful day and avoid self-harming without eating any meals or snacks. The research on self-regulation suggests that curbing impulses is associated with levels of glucose metabolism in the brain, leading some researchers to conclude that glucose is an important biological fuel for self-regulation (Gailliot & Baumeister, 2007; Kurzban, 2010; cf. Beedie & Lane, 2011). These are just a couple of examples of how a clinician might use knowledge from behavioral science to convey the likely consequence of a client's behavior.

The clinician also can use a case formulation to guide predictions about the likely consequences of client behavior. In the example of the client who was terrified of an upcoming job interview, the clinician might know from previous assessment that, when the client uses the skill of opposite action and confidently approaches difficult conversations, he feels less anxious and performs quite well. In contrast, when he cancels or avoids situations like job interviews, he often feels guilty and ashamed. The clinician might remind the client of these contingencies. Finally, sometimes the likely consequences of the client's behavior are obvious. The client, for example, who uses the DBT interpersonal effectiveness skills of DEAR MAN while yelling at his partner is likely to get a less desirable response then he would if he were to use a more gentle approach (i.e., the GIVE skills; Linehan, 1993b, 2015).

Characteristics of Feedback

Other important considerations have to do with the characteristics of the clinician's feedback, including its timing, density, and specificity (Farmer & Chapman, 2016). In terms of *timing,* feedback occurring close in time to the occurrence of the client's behavior is more likely to be effective than delayed feedback. *Density* of feedback has to do with how much feedback the clinician provides. Particularly when a distressed client calls for skills coaching, or when the client is in the skill acquisition phase, it can be effective for the clinician to make a couple of suggestions on how the client can use the skill more effectively. Overly elaborate or dense feedback can be overwhelming, and the client might be likely to forget or miss key points (Farmer & Chapman, 2016).

In terms of *specificity,* there has been some debate regarding whether detailed or general feedback is more effective (see also Follette & Callaghan, 1995, for a discussion of issues pertaining to specific versus general feedback in the training of clinicians). Detailed feedback involves comments on the specific ways in which the client has used a skill. The clinician above provided detailed feedback on the client's use of paced breathing. While it is often easier and perhaps more desirable to provide specific versus general feedback during skills coaching, one risk is that specific feedback might encourage rule-governed behavior and reduce the client's ability to flexibly use skills according to varying contextual demands (Farmer & Chapman, 2016).

In contrast with specific feedback, general feedback might involve simply conveying that the behavior was effective or ineffective. It is up to the client, then, to figure out how to improve. In martial arts training, I've sometimes found general feedback to be helpful. When an instructor says that I did something well but does not specify what I did, this gives me the opportunity to figure it out myself. Thinking through how I used a particular strategy improves my ability to reflect and self-correct over time. Similarly, a clinician might tell the client above that he did a great job asking the roommate for space, without specifying what the client did well. To take this a step further, the clinician might ask the client what he thought he did well. When I supervise students in therapy, I often review video- or audio-recordings of portions of therapy sessions. Following this review, I often ask the student what she thought she did well and what could have been improved. Ultimately, I want my supervisees to become their own supervisors, just as I would like my clients to become their own therapists. Therefore, given enough time, this approach can be helpful in skills coaching with clients. Clinicians should seek to find the most effective way to give feedback, given the client's unique skills and circumstances.

Being Dialectical about Skills Coaching

There are a few key dialectics to consider regarding skills coaching. One dialectic is between the client's current capabilities and the capabilities the client will need to build to develop a life worth living. The clinician must titrate her approach to skills coaching to the client's current capabilities, using principles of shaping, and keep the ultimate goal in mind. Consider a client, for example, who is anxious, avoids other people, and has social skill deficits but desperately wants more emotionally intimate relationships. The clinician will need to have reasonable expectations regarding the client's ability to use interpersonal skills to hold a conversation and find ways to scaffold these skills to help the client engage with others in more sophisticated and emotionally intimate ways. In DBT, we assume that clients are both doing the best they can *and* need to do better in order to develop a life worth living. A second, key dialectic is that of specific versus general feedback. Clients often need very specific feedback to understand how to use a skill, and when the clinician provides such specific feedback, the client may not learn to think the situation through on his or her own. Similarly, when I edit graduate students' papers, if I rewrite sentences, my students are likely to mindlessly accept the changes and unlikely to learn what was wrong with the sentence in the first place. Therefore, I recommend that the clinician provide specific feedback when needed and seek ways to help the client develop the ability to think through dilemmas and difficult situations and consider what skills to use and how to use them. Finally, a third dialectic that cuts across all of DBT is that of acceptance and change. Skills coaching is a change-oriented strategy, as the clinician is trying to help the client change her behavior and use effective skills to navigate difficult situations. Without first accepting the client and her current capabilities, emotional experiences, and situation, the clinician is unlikely to provide helpful skills coaching. The clinician must often practice acceptance of the client and convey this acceptance through validation, which can balance the change-oriented focus of skills coaching. As mentioned earlier, it is also helpful to balance suggestions for the client to use acceptance and change-oriented skills.

Summary

In summary, phone coaching (and skills coaching more broadly) involves a few core strategies. As mentioned in the previous chapter, an initial step in phone coaching is to assess the problem prompting the phone call. In a similar way, during the coaching phase of the call, the clinician also often starts with an assessment of the client's difficulties in using skills. Following this assessment, the clinician provides instructions to use certain skills or tips on how to use skills more effectively. It can be very effective to prompt the client to try out the skill and to observe (or assesses through asking questions) the client's behavior. Close observation of the client's use of a skill helps the clinician to provide useful feedback. Following this feedback, the clinician often provides further instruction and/or prompts the client to incorporate the clinician's feedback and try the skill again. Time permitting, the cycle may continue until the client is able to use the skill effectively. Time, however, is often short during phone coaching; thus, the clinician may not always use all of the strategies above or in the order in which they were presented.

Notwithstanding, it is important for clinicians to remember that DBT (and CBT more broadly) is more of a "doing" therapy than a "talking" therapy. As such, in phone coaching, as in therapy or skills sessions, it is more effective for the clinician to activate or "drag out" new behavior. Doing so allows the clinician to assess the client's proficiency with skills and to provide accurate feedback. Finally, it is useful for clinicians to tailor their approach to skills coaching to the client's stage of learning (skill acquisition, strengthening, or generalization). Some examples in this chapter were included to show how a clinician might take a different approach to clients in the skill acquisition versus strengthening phase. Chapter 9 devotes further attention to ways to help clients generalize their skills to different contexts and beyond therapy. Now that I have covered standard structural (Chapter 4) and skills-coaching strategies (the present chapter), in the next chapter, I focus on core DBT skills to help clients regulate and tolerate emotions.

CHAPTER 6

Coaching in Emotion Regulation and Distress Tolerance

C lients often call for help with stressful situations ranging from interpersonal conflicts, to problems with extremely intense emotional states, to urges to engage in aggressive behavior toward oneself or others, and so on. Although clinicians cannot be experts in all possible skills related to these situations, maintaining awareness of the primary goals of phone coaching can help the clinician to zero-in on the most effective, immediately useful skills. Often the best that can be done in the time available for a phone coaching call (or a quick coaching session in a milieu or individual or group treatment) is to help clients avoid worsening difficult situations and use their skills to tolerate or regulate emotional reactions in these situations until something changes. In DBT, there are four primary sets of skills: mindfulness, interpersonal effectiveness, emotion regulation (ER), and distress tolerance (Linehan, 1993b, 2015). Beyond DBT skills, other forms of CBT include a variety of additional coping, interpersonal, and other skills. Clinicians cannot be expected to have developed expertise in all possible skills. The focus of this chapter is on selected ER and distress tolerance skills, as these are perhaps the most commonly used skills during phone coaching. This chapter begins with a discussion of emotions and ER and then includes a review of particularly helpful skills in the areas of ER and distress tolerance, along with case vignettes to illustrate phone coaching on these skills. The focus is on skills that the clinician can easily and quickly coach the client on during phone coaching calls. Readers who wish to learn more about the gamut of DBT skills should read the *DBT Skills Training Manual, 2nd Edition* (Linehan, 2015).

Emotions and Emotion Regulation

DBT is an emotion-focused therapy. The biosocial theory underlying the treatment posits that BPD results from a transaction of a biological, temperamental vulnerability to emotions with an invalidating rearing environment (Crowell et al., 2009; Linehan, 1993a). The individual at risk of developing BPD has an emotional temperament characterized by emotional sensitivity (low threshold for emotional arousal), reactivity (intense emotional responses), and slow return to emotional baseline (delayed recovery to baseline emotional arousal). The invalidating environment, ranging from a poor fit with the child's temperament to environments characterized by trauma, abuse, and neglect, (1) rejects the child's communication of private experiences (emotions, thoughts, etc.) regardless of their validity, (2) oversimplifies the ease of solving problems or overcoming stressors, and (3) intermittently reinforces intense emotional communication (Linehan, 1993a). The child's temperament and the invalidating environment transact, such that each factor intensifies the other. Invalidation amplifies emotional arousal and dysregulation, and dysregulated emotions set the stage for further invalidation, and so forth. The child does not learn to effectively understand, label, regulate, or communicate emotions, and this fundamental deficit in ER often cuts across the many interpersonal and behavioral problems experienced by people with BPD (and often, those with other complex mental health problems).

As an emotion-focused therapy, many interventions and skills in DBT aim to help the client learn to understand, regulate, and effectively communicate emotions. DBT includes ER skills designed to help clients learn to understand and effectively regulate emotions; interpersonal effectiveness skills to effectively express needs, communicate, and enhance relationships; emotional exposure strategies to help clients experience, tolerate, and reduce fear of emotions; among several other interventions. Similarly, in phone coaching, the primary goal often is to help the client regulate or tolerate overwhelming emotions.

Given the emotion-focused nature of DBT more broadly and phone coaching specifically, it is helpful for the clinician to have a working knowledge of emotions and ER. My favorite definition of ER is that of James Gross (1998): "the ways in which we influence which emotions we have, when we have them, and how we experience and express them." Indeed, helping the client use skills to understand, experience, modify, or express emotions is often a key goal of phone coaching.

To accomplish this goal, it is helpful to understand how emotions work. A clear ER also can help the clinician respond effectively when the client is experiencing or expressing emotions that make phone coaching challenging. Below, I discuss some of the key components of emotions and how understanding these components can facilitate phone coaching. I would highly recommend that clinicians conducting phone coaching consider further reading on the field of ER. One helpful, comprehensive resource on ER is the *Handbook of Emotion Regulation, Second Edition* (Gross, 2015).

Although it would be difficult to arrive at a definition of emotions that everyone in the field would agree on, emerging consensus suggests that emotions have several key features. Emotions tend to (1) be multifaceted, (2) occur in motivationally relevant situations, and (3) are related to characteristic action tendencies. The discussion below addresses these key components and how they relate to phone coaching (and skills coaching more broadly).

Emotions are Multifaceted

Emotions tend to be multifaceted, consisting of many parts or components. When an emotional response occurs, changes occur in physiological and neurological activity, subjective experience, urges to engage in particular actions, cognition, and behavior. In this way, an emotional response can be conceptualized broadly as a collection of physiological, cognitive, and behavioral activities. These activities tend to occur closely in time. Fear, for example, may consist of a combination of increased activity in the limbic system of the brain; activation of the hypothalamic–adrenal–pituitary axis, resulting in increased cortisol secretion; subjective sensations of increased body temperature, muscle tension, and heart rate; narrowed attention and cognition; and the activation of behavioral tendencies toward flight, fight, or freeze responses. Other emotions have different physiological, cognitive, and behavioral profiles.

Understanding that emotions have physiological, cognitive, and behavioral features can help clinicians to effectively coach clients in ways to regulate emotions. While research has found that these three broad components of emotions are not always as highly correlated as they seem (this is why some researchers have framed the components of emotions as "loosely coupled"; see Gross, 2015), changes in one component can often result in changes in other components. When a client, for example, calls for help in coping with intense sadness, she or he may be struggling primarily with overwhelming subjective sensations of sadness and difficulty tolerating sadness-related thoughts. Yet, changing the *behavioral* component of sadness is often the most effective ER strategy. Coaching might, therefore, focus on ways to help the client activate behaviors that run counter to sadness, such as engaging in stimulating or pleasurable activities and spending time or seeking support from others. Alternatively, the clinician might coach the client to mindfully experience and accept the physiological sensations of sadness (using the skill of mindfulness of current emotion, discussed below). Because of the multifaceted nature of emotions, there are "many roads to Rome" (i.e., many pathways to effective ER). I often tell clients that one of the things I love about emotions is that they have different components. Changing one component can change the whole emotion.

Emotions Tend to Occur in Motivationally Relevant Situations

Another key feature is that emotions tend to occur in situations that we perceive as relevant to our goals (Mauss & Tamir, 2013)—what some have described as *motivationally relevant* situations (Gross, 2015; Ochsner & Gross, 2015). This means that emotions arise in situations that have some bearing on factors that are important to us. A bomb threat, for example, is likely to elicit fear because this situation would be perceived as a threat to our goals of safety and survival. Sadness is a common reaction to loss including the loss of loved ones, relationships, or even important aspirations. This is probably because such losses thwart needs (to be connected with loved ones) or goals (to make certain achievements) that are important to us.

When strong emotions arise, some aspect of the situation (or how the client perceives it) is often relevant to goals or needs that are important to the client. A client calling for phone coaching following a relationship conflict might feel sad and angry because the conflict impedes his goal to be supported and connected. Phone coaching, therefore, might focus on short-term strategies to increase connection and seek support, perhaps incorporating interpersonal skills (to ask others for help or seek out contact with others). As another example, one of our clients became suicidal and called the clinician toward the end of treatment and was having a hard time with hopeless thoughts, frustration, and sadness. His psychiatrist recently had retired, and he was sad about this loss and worried he would be left without adequate psychiatric care following the end of therapy. In the short term, phone coaching involved distress tolerance skills to reduce suicide risk, self-soothe, and distract; and in the next session, the clinician helped the client use problem-solving skills (see Linehan, 2015) to work through barriers to his goal of having psychiatric care.

Emotions Are Related to Characteristic Action Tendencies

One implication of the motivationally relevant nature of emotions is that they are our body and brain's way of alerting us to important situations that we may need to pay attention to or do something about. This is probably why emotions are so closely linked to specific action tendencies. When an emotion signals that something important might be happening, it is common to feel the desire (referred to in DBT as an *action urge*; Linehan, 2015) to engage in one of a couple of broad categories of behavior: approach or avoid. Certain emotions are commonly related to approach tendencies, such as when anger or frustration sparks the desire to move forward, fight injustice, get around barriers, and solve problems. In contrast, other emotions such as fear or sadness often are related to avoidance tendencies, such as to escape or withdraw. Complex emotional states, such as shame (where behavioral tendencies often consist of hiding and/or appeasing/atoning) or rapidly occurring mixed emotions, might result in conflicts between behavioral tendencies toward approach or avoidance.

Understanding that emotions are related to motivationally relevant situations and spur action tendencies can help clinicians to effectively navigate phone coaching with clients who are experiencing strong emotions. When a client describes an overwhelming emotion, it can be helpful to try to understand what aspect of the triggering situation is relevant to the client's needs or goals: What about this situation (or about the client's thoughts about this situation) is important enough to trigger a strong emotional reaction? As discussed below in the section on opposite action, sometimes, while the emotional reaction is understandable, it is a false alarm. The client may experience the situation as a threat to her or his goals, when no actual threat is present. At other times, the emotional response might be a true alarm, in that the emotion fits the current situation.

As emotions are tightly linked with action tendencies, I also seek to understand what the client feels like doing in the presence of the strong emotion. Indeed, one of the most effective ER strategies involves engaging in behavior that opposes the action tendencies associated with the emotion. In DBT, this is the skill of *opposite action*. Other contemporary forms of CBT have also emphasized the importance of reversing action tendencies related to emotions (e.g., the Unified Protocol for Emotional Disorders; see Barlow, 2011).

Emotions Often Function to Communicate

Research and theory also suggest that emotions evolved partly to facilitate survival by encouraging social and group bonds. One mechanism for these bonds is the communication of danger, important information, intentions, and needs (LeDoux, 2002; Quinlan & Quinlan, 2007). As such, emotion-linked action tendencies often include communicating or expressing feelings, wishes, and desires. Understanding that emotions often spur the need to express or communicate can be very useful in phone coaching and in therapy more broadly. Many clinicians have encountered the situation in which their clients (or loved ones!) continue to repeat the same statements with increasing intensity. I have found anecdotally that this often occurs when the clinician has not adequately expressed understanding of the client's experiences or perspective. Often, emotions simply need to be communicated. Once it is clear that the message has gotten through to another person, the emotional experience diminishes. This is probably why accurate validation has such a strong emotion-regulating effect (Fruzzetti & Shenk, 2008). In phone coaching, then, the challenge is sometimes for the clinician to be able to quickly, concisely, and accurately validate the client's experiences.

Stepping back, observing the client's reactions, and engaging in accurate validation sometimes requires acceptance and patience. I once saw a client who taught me a lot about acceptance and patience during phone coaching. Knowing that the main goal of phone coaching is to coach the client on the effective use of skills, I approached coaching calls with this client in a very goal-directed manner. I wanted to get down to business, quickly understand the situation, and help him figure out how to use helpful skills. The client, however, kept talking over me, rejecting my suggestions, and repeatedly describing the stressful situations he was experiencing. I felt increasingly frustrated and time-pressured, and tried even harder to get down to business. You can imagine how this backfired! The client kept talking longer about how upset he was and seemed unwilling to talk about skills. We were polarized, and our calls were long and painful. With some help from my DBT consultation team, I decided to try a different approach. I still structured the coaching call in the manner described in Chapter 3, but I decided to spend the first 3 or 4 minutes stepping back, paying attention to the client's experience, and trying to understand what was going on before discussing skills. I tried to let go of my desire to move things along really quickly, and paradoxically letting go of being efficient made our calls much more efficient! When the client felt understood, he stopped repeating himself and seemed much more open to my suggestions regarding skills. As much as I emphasize to trainees that skills coaching should focus on skills, it's just as important to remember that anyone experiencing extremely intense emotions probably first needs to feel heard and understood.

Coaching on Key Emotion Regulation Skills

ER skills in DBT are comprehensive (Linehan, 1993a, 2015). Clients typically are first provided with psychoeducation on the nature of emotions and the functions that emotions serve in our lives, as well as tips on how to label emotions. Some ER skills involve reducing vulnerability to stress and overwhelming emotions, and others target situations (problem solving) or thinking patterns (checking the facts) associated with unwanted emotions. The DBT ER skills also include behavioral strategies to modify action tendencies associated with particular emotions (i.e., opposite action). I could spend this whole book and more discussing ways to coach clients in the various ER skills, but I decided to focus here on two ER skills that are especially helpful during brief phone coaching calls: mindfulness of current emotion and opposite action.

Mindfulness of Current Emotions

The skill of *mindfulness of current emotions* involves nonjudgmentally observing and experiencing an emotional state. Clients are taught to attend closely to the bodily sensations associated with the emotion and to avoid escaping, blocking, suppressing, or attempting to maintain the emotional experience. When thoughts, judgments, urges, and so on arise, the idea is to let these experiences go and redirect attention back to the sensations of the emotion. Clients learn to ride out an intense emotional state like a wave on the ocean, noticing as the emotion peaks and crests, falls, and rises again. When practicing this skill, it is important to avoid acting on the emotion itself. In addition, clients are taught that they are *not* their emotion. Their emotion is an experience they are having, but there is more to them than that emotional experience. Over time, this skill can help the client learn how to tolerate her or his emotions and gain practice in avoiding acting on impulses-associated emotions (e.g., the urge to yell, to lash out, to harm oneself). As this skill can be particularly helpful when clients call experiencing overwhelming or intense emotions, I often coach skills in mindfulness of current emotion during phone coaching.

There are a few key points to keep in mind when coaching clients on this skill. First, mindfulness of current emotions is one of several skills designed to help clients cope with extremely intense emotions. This skill, therefore, is often quite helpful when a client calls for help coping with very intense emotions. Although mindfulness of current emotions can be helpful anytime, a client's extreme emotional expression is a cue that this skill might be particularly helpful.

Second, this skill can be particularly helpful when clients appear to be avoiding or escaping their emotions. A certain degree of avoidance or escape, of course, can be useful to ride out crisis situations (and is encouraged in some of the distress tolerance skills), but DBT and other forms of CBT generally aim to help clients move away from emotional avoidance. When a client shows signs of emotional avoidance (e.g., avoiding certain topics, changing the subject, showing a disconnect between affect and the content of the conversation) during phone coaching, the clinician might consider coaching the client to focus on her or his current physiological sensations of emotions. Thinking patterns, such as worry or rumination, also can sometimes be considered escape behavior; thus, it can be helpful to guide the client to redirect her or his attention to the current emotion. In addition, clients (and clinicians) sometimes take an imbalanced approach to skills, erring on the side of skills to change or distract from emotions. Mindfulness of current emotion fits the acceptance end of the dialectic and can help balance out the predominantly change-oriented approach that many clients take when they are particularly upset.

Third, as mentioned in an earlier case example, mindfulness does not involve pushing away, ignoring, or getting rid of experiences. Clients and clinicians alike often have the misconception that mindfulness involves ignoring, pushing away, or getting rid of distracting or distressing thoughts. I have often heard clinicians in my team meetings say they had a hard time getting away from their thoughts during the mindfulness exercise. This is not the point of mindfulness. Upsetting memories, thoughts, urges, images, and so on may arise during any mindfulness practice. The goal is not to ignore, push away, avoid, or get rid of these experiences. Rather, the practice of mindfulness involves noticing distracting experiences and gently guiding one's mind back to the experience of the present moment. In the case of mindfulness of current emotion, the client's focus is on her or his sensations of the emotional state.

Finally, sometimes clients are reluctant to use this skill out of fear of their emotions or concerns that the emotion will last for an excessive or interminable period. Under these circumstances, it is helpful to remind clients that emotional states are time-limited, usually lasting seconds to minutes at most (Ekman, 1999). Mindful observation with a spirit of curiosity will allow the emotions to run their course. I often tell clients that our emotions would usually simply run their course if we were to stop messing with them. I define "messing with them" as worrying, ruminating, trying to escape or avoid, acting on them, and so forth. In addition, it can be helpful to remind clients who are afraid of experiencing their emotions that, over time, mindfulness of current emotion will help them overcome this fear. Fear of emotions is often related to past learning, whereby the presence of an emotional state has become paired with some kind of negative occurrence. A client who is afraid of experiencing sadness might, for example, have a learning history whereby expressions of sadness were met with severe invalidation, punishment, or abuse. Over time, sadness has become associated with threatening events. Much like exposure therapy, mindfulness of current sadness in the absence of threatening events would be expected to help the client develop new, nonthreatening associations with sadness.

CLIENT: Alice, I just don't know what to do right now, I'm going crazy. [*client is breathing quickly, and his voice is loud and high-pitched*] I . . . I . . .

THERAPIST: John, you're having a really hard time. I'm going to ask you to slow down a bit, and tell me what's happening.

CLIENT: I don't know if I can. I can't think. I just. . . . Oh, my God!

THERAPIST: OK, start with breathing, John. Don't say anything for about a minute. Just focus on your breathing. Slow everything down. Take a slow breath with me, and slowly exhale. Inhale . . . exhale.

CLIENT: [inhales and exhales for about 30 seconds to a minute]

THERAPIST: Now, describe what's happening and what you're feeling.

CLIENT: I'm just freaking out. I don't know why I was so stupid. I was at a party last night, and I guess I had way too much to drink. I don't know, I woke up with Joanie, and I don't think I used any protection or anything. She's HIV-positive! What have I done?! [breathing quickly and shallowly] I don't know what to do.

THERAPIST: That sounds really scary, John. We'll figure out what you can do. Right now, I want you to slow everything down, and go back to your breathing. Now, focus on your emotions and where you're feeling them in your body.

CLIENT: [breathing more slowly] I feel, like, this sick sensation in my stomach. I'm so scared!

THERAPIST: Come back to your body. Sick sensation in your stomach. . . .

CLIENT: Yeah, and my arms are really tight. My chest feels like this adrenaline surge or something.

THERAPIST: OK, let's take a minute and have you just notice your sensations. This is mindfulness of your emotion. I think this is going to help you so that we can talk about what to do from here.

CLIENT: OK, I'll try.

THERAPIST: Just keep your mind on your sensations. Ride the wave. If thoughts come, gently let them go, and come back to your body.

CLIENT: [after a couple of minutes] OK, I think I can talk now, but I'm still pretty freaked out. I can't believe I did this. What am I going to do?

THERAPIST: OK, I know, this is really hard. You feel just sick about the possibilities. Let's just talk about a couple of steps you can take between now and Thursday when we meet. . . . [They talk about steps to take.]

THERAPIST: OK, I think we've got a good plan for steps you can take between now and Thursday. In the meantime, remember your distress tolerance plan for this evening. Your job is to just get through the evening without making anything worse. If emotions go through the roof, start with mindfulness like we did on the phone, and then if you need to, try the TIP skills. They've often worked pretty well for you, right?

CLIENT: Yeah, I can do that, I already have a bowl in the fridge with cold water just in case!

In this example, the client called in a panic about the possibility of HIV, and the therapist guided him in mindfulness of current emotion. The client was able to use this skill to ride the wave of fear and get to the point where he could talk. In this situation, clearly, mindfulness of current emotion would not be the only skill to use. The client likely will have to use problem-solving strategies to determine the next steps to address his fears, and some of those steps might involve making an appointment with his physician, discussing when and how to get lab tests for HIV, coming up with a plan to have appropriate support people available, and so forth. During phone coaching, I find it helpful just to focus on the next logical step, such as making an appointment with the physician, rather than to entertain the gamut of steps between the current situation and a lifetime regimen of antiretroviral medications. When clients are in emotion mind and feeling overwhelmed, it's often best to focus on one thing in the moment (one of the distress tolerance skills).

Opposite Action

Opposite action involves engaging in actions that oppose the action tendencies associated with a particular emotion. Clients are taught to identify their specific emotional state and the action urge associated with that emotional state. An *action urge* is the desire to engage in a particular type of behavior (Linehan, 1993b, 2015). As mentioned earlier, one of the primary adaptive features of emotions is that they compel actions that help us reach goals. As such, emotions often come along with urges to engage in particular types of behavior. Anger and frustration, for example, are often associated with action urges to engage in some form of aggressive behavior. In contrast, fear and anxiety are associated with action urges to avoid, escape, or scan the environment for danger. When an emotional state accurately fits a particular situation, it often is effective to act on the action urge. If I were feeling afraid in the presence of a pit viper, it would be effective to act on my urge to get out of the situation (but carefully).

In the context of sadness regarding the loss of a significant other, action urges might compel us to take care of ourselves and seek support.

Opposite action is not typically used in these situations in which the emotional state fits the facts of the current situation. Instead, opposite action is most effective when the emotional state does *not* fit the current situation. If a client, for example, was afraid that he would be humiliated if he spoke up in class, his fear would not fit most classroom situations (unless he disrobed and asked the teacher to marry him). Doing what he feels like doing (escaping, avoiding, cancelling his class, skipping class on the day of his presentation—all of which I've done in the past by the way!) prevents him from learning that his fears will not come true. Opposite action in this situation would involve attending class, confidently speaking up, enthusiastically giving his class presentation, and so on. Much like exposure therapy for fear- or anxiety-related disorders, over time, opposite action in this situation would be expected to help the client learn that it is safe to speak up in class, and that fear can be tolerated.

In other cases, however, opposite action might be helpful even if the emotion fits the situation. Most commonly, this is the case for anger- or frustration-related emotions. Linehan (2015) has made the point that anger is often justifiable based on the current situation; the problem is that anger often compels ineffective behavior, such as yelling or acting aggressively. As a result, even if their anger-related emotions are justifiable, it can still be effective for clients to do the opposite of what their anger is telling them to do. Some common opposite actions for anger include gently avoiding the object of anger (person or situation), trying to engender empathy or compassion toward someone else, and perspective taking. Engaging in behavior that opposes the action urge often dampens the experience of anger. Over time, the client may learn to act effectively even when she or he is angry.

I encourage clinicians to try out this skill as well as many of the others detailed in Linehan's (2015) skills training manual. I believe that practicing the skills we coach can make us better coaches. I was recently in a situation in which I believed I was being treated unfairly and felt quite frustrated and angry. Even though I did not want to, I tried out the skill of opposite action by taking the perspective of the person or people involved. I found that, fairly quickly, my anger and frustration reduced. What I found most interesting was that a sense of sadness about the situation took the place of the anger. After a few practices of experiencing the sadness mindfully, I started to feel more free of my anger, tension, and resentment, even though I was regularly reminded of the situation. Clients' experiences will not always be consistent with my own, but knowing that this is sometimes what happens when opposite action for anger is practiced can be helpful.

Clinical Example of Coaching on Mindfulness of Current Emotion and Opposite Action

In the example below, the client calls and expresses distress regarding a recent interaction with an old friend. She has been having suicidal thoughts but has committed not to do anything to harm herself. The excerpt begins after the clinician has used some of the structural strategies occurring at the beginning of phone coaching calls (see Chapter 4). Because of space limitations, I have not presented structural strategies for the ending of the call. I would, however, encourage the reader to write a complete script for an excerpt of her or his own that involves coaching a client on key ER skills (see Exercise 6.1).

THERAPIST: Just so I'm clearer on the problem, you've been having a really hard time since you met up with your old friend.

CLIENT: Yeah, I mean I've just been having so many feelings, and I don't know what to do. She recently got married. She also got promoted at work. All of that's just so far beyond me. I'm just stuck at home with my dad, and I can't even get myself out to do volunteer work. I don't know if I'll ever meet someone.

THERAPIST: It can be really hard to be reminded that you're not where you really want to be. What emotions have been coming up for you?

CLIENT: Well, I don't really resent her. She's a good friend, and I want her to be happy, but I don't know, I guess it's jealousy.

THERAPIST: That sounds about right. Maybe it's more like envy. Envy comes up when someone else has something important to you that you don't have. Does that sound right?

CLIENT: Yeah, it does. I mean, why do I have to be the one with all these mental health problems, while she just sails along so easily? I don't know, I just don't see any point in going on when it's always so hard for me. It's just going to keep being hard, and I don't think I have it in me to keep going.

THERAPIST: The envy makes a lot of sense to me, and I know you've often felt like you can't keep up this struggle. I also know it has already gotten easier, and I'm confident we can keep chipping away at this misery so it doesn't have to be so hard all the time. Have you had suicidal thoughts?

CLIENT: Yeah, I mean, I just don't see the point.

THERAPIST: I'm guessing that you wouldn't be thinking of suicide if you weren't dealing with such painful emotions. What emotion would you say is most related to the suicidal thoughts? What emotion are you having the hardest time with? The envy or the sadness, or something else?

CLIENT: I think it's the sadness. I just feel so sad that I'll never have the kind of life I want.

THERAPIST: Sadness that you don't have the life you really want makes a lot of sense. I'm not so sure about sadness that you'll never have it. The thought that you'll never have it sounds like hopelessness. We don't know if you'll never have it; we just know that you don't have it now.

CLIENT: I guess, but I really just don't see how I'll ever get there . . .

THERAPIST: We're going to keep working on it, and I have faith that we'll get there. I know it's hard to see right now, though. Here's what I think would help—remember the skill of opposite action?

CLIENT: Doing the opposite of what I feel like doing?

THERAPIST: Exactly.

CLIENT: But I thought I read in my binder that opposite action is just for times when my emotion isn't accurate or something.

THERAPIST: Nice catch, Cheryl! You've been doing your homework. Usually, that's true. But I still think it could be helpful here. Would you say that most of the sadness is related to your hopeless thoughts or to the way your life is right now?

CLIENT: I guess it's more the hopeless thoughts. I mean, I normally feel a little sad about the way things are, but not this sad. This is crazy!

THERAPIST: Hmmm. Crazy is a judgment, but I'll let that one go for now. I think we're onto something. Sadness about a bad future that you're imagining doesn't fit the facts. You're not in that future. You're here. We really have no idea what your future holds, so you're feeling sad about something that might not even happen, not if I can help it!

That's why I think opposite action would help. What are the sadness and hopelessness making you feel like doing right now?

CLIENT: Well, I called because of the suicide urges, but for the record, I'm not planning to act on them. I know we have our agreement. I just, I guess I feel like giving up on that stupid volunteering application. Maybe just curling up, staying in my room, and just going to sleep.

THERAPIST: Is it close to your bedtime?

CLIENT: Hey, it's 2: 00 P.M. Come on!

THERAPIST: Stranger things have happened. I seem to remember you staying in bed for most of the afternoon not too long ago. In any case, what's one thing you could do that's the opposite of what your hopeless thoughts and sadness are telling you to do? If you want to stay in, give up, and do nothing . . .

CLIENT: I guess the opposite would be to get back to work on the application.

THERAPIST: That sounds wise. You could take small steps. Do what you'd do if you had more hope. But I'm thinking it might be good to combine that with getting out. Let's have you go opposite to the urge to just stay in your room. We know where that normally takes you.

CLIENT: OK, but where would I go?

THERAPIST: Maybe someplace where you can work on your application? How about the library? You've been walking there regularly.

CLIENT: True, I could get myself to go to the library. It's not far, and it's quiet . . .

THERAPIST: OK, good plan. I think we might be missing something, though.

CLIENT: What?

THERAPIST: Well, if you have a wave of sadness that's about the way your life is right now, it might be worth practicing mindfulness of current emotion.

CLIENT: Why would I want to do that?

THERAPIST: Kind of like we've discussed before, sadness can be a really helpful emotion to experience and learn from. Sadness about an imagined bad future isn't so helpful, but sadness about your current life might be telling you something needs to change. As an

EXERCISE 6.1 Writing Excerpts/Scripts for Coaching on Key Emotion Regulation Skills

Writing out a script of what you might say or do can be excellent practice for phone coaching regarding particular skills. Consider a client you are working with or have worked with in the past. Think about the type of problem that would prompt a call from this client. On a separate piece of paper or in a word-processing document, write out a script, from start to finish, showing how you would navigate a phone coaching call, focusing on key ER skills, such as opposite action and/ or mindfulness of current emotion.

experiment, I'd like to suggest that you try out mindfulness of that sadness for about 5–10 minutes or so, and then try the opposite action of going to the library. What do you think?

In this example, the clinician assessed the factors related to the client's emotional experiences, zeroing in on sadness and envy. The clinician also assessed which emotion seems most related to suicidality, and when the client reported sadness, the focus was on skills to manage sadness. The important and perhaps subtle distinction in this example was between the kind of sadness that was justified (sadness about her life not being the way she wanted it to be) and the kind of sadness that was potentially unjustified (sadness as a reaction to hopeless thoughts about the future). In terms of skills-coaching suggestions, the clinician combined opposite action and mindfulness of sadness related to the current state of the client's life.

Coaching on Key Distress Tolerance Skills

Distress tolerance skills include strategies for clients to ride out painful or difficult situations or emotions without making their problems worse, until they can find some way to improve the situation. Clients are taught strategies to get through a crisis, to accept reality as it is, and to engage in effective action. Crisis survival strategies are particularly helpful in riding out urges to engage in dysfunctional behaviors (e.g., self-injury, suicidal behavior); thus, they often are among the most helpful go-to skills during phone coaching. Crisis survival skills include strategies to avoid engaging in unwise or impulsive actions (i.e., the "STOP" skill; Linehan, 2015); increase motivation to tolerate distress (by considering pros and cons); distract themselves from difficult situations, thoughts, and feelings (the "ACCEPTS" skills); engage in self-soothing; and make each moment more bearable (the "IMPROVE" the moment skills). Other crisis survival skills (the TIP skills) are particularly helpful in the event of extremely intense emotions that interfere with the client's ability to think about or solve problems.

Key Points in Coaching on Distress Tolerance Skills

There are at least three key points to keep in mind when coaching clients on crisis survival strategies. First, crisis survival strategies will not solve the problem leading to a crisis. Clients sometimes report that the crisis survival skills they were taught did not work, partly because the problem did not go away. During skills training or phone coaching, therefore, it is helpful to let clients know that these skills will not solve their problems. A client won't solve a relationship conflict by taking a time-out and soothing his or her anger, but he or she will avoid yelling, screaming, or otherwise making things worse. Longer-term work can be done in therapy to solve and prevent problems precipitating crises or reduce misery.

Second, crisis survival strategies can be considered successful if the client has avoided problematic behavior. Even if the client did not feel better during or after using these strategies, the skills were still successful if she or he avoided harmful behavior. Clients sometimes are dissatisfied with crisis survival skills, reporting that they did not feel better while using them, or that they felt only temporary relief. A client, for example, distracting himself from painful emotions by watching television, might find that these emotions return shortly after the television goes off. This is to be expected. Crisis survival skills take the edge off or distract the client from painful emotions but do not generally solve the problem or result in long-term relief. The skills have "worked" if (1) the client could tolerate her or his emotional pain while using the skills and (2) the client avoided engaging in problematic or harmful behavior.

Third, crisis survival skills work best when clients use them mindfully. If a client using distraction is not paying attention to the distracting activity or is ruminating or worrying about a distressing problem, distraction may not result in noticeable relief. Even if harmful behavior is avoided, the lack of relief might make the client reluctant to keep using the skill. Coaching on the use of crisis survival skills, therefore, often involves encouraging the client to use these skills mindfully.

Clinical Example of Coaching on Distress Tolerance Skills

In the example below, the client, Sam, calls after a conflict in which his partner discovers that Sam previously slept with another woman. He is extremely upset but has not yet tried any skills.

THERAPIST: Hi, Sam. I should let you know that I've got about 10 minutes or so. Why don't you give me a short description of the problem that led you to call?

CLIENT: OK, this is a big one, though. I don't know what to do. My girlfriend found some e-mails from when I slept with someone else. I mean, it was so minor, just like a one-night stand, but she's really, really upset, and she says she's not sure she can stay with me anymore. She packed up and left for the night. I just feel so sick and scared, and I don't know what to do. I mean, I know I messed up, but I don't want to lose her. I was thinking of asking her to marry me.

THERAPIST: Oh, Sam, I'm so sorry to hear this. I know how much Julie means to you. I'm glad you called, and think we can help you get through this until we meet on Tuesday. What skills have you tried so far?

CLIENT: Oh, I don't know, nothing really. I can't really think, and I don't know what to do. I just picked up the phone.

THERAPIST: I'm sure it's hard to think right now with how upset you are. Do you know where your skills binder is?

CLIENT: Yeah, it's in my room.

THERAPIST: OK, here's what I'd like you to do. Get off the phone, and go and flip through to the sections on self-soothing and the TIP skills. Try out a couple of those, and we can talk later if you need to.

CLIENT: OK, I'll give it a try.

In this example, Sam had called before trying out any skills. This is understandable, given how upset he is, but the clinician ideally should maintain the expectation that the client will try skills before calling (see Chapter 3). Clients often call when they are upset, and if the clinician decides whether to enforce this expectation based on how upset the client is, she or he risks reinforcing the client's use of phone coaching in the absence of skills practice. In the example below, Sam calls the clinician back after having tried some distress tolerance skills.

THERAPIST: Hi, Sam, what have you tried so far?

CLIENT: Well, I tried some of the self-soothing stuff. I usually really like that TV channel that shows photos and stuff from around the world, so I watched that for a while, and I listened to some music.

THERAPIST: How did that work?

CLIENT: It really didn't work.

THERAPIST: Oh, what do you mean by that?

CLIENT: I kind of felt a little better while I was watching TV, but it only lasted for a little while, and I started to have a really hard time again. That's why I listened to the music, but that didn't work at all.

THERAPIST: Did you do anything drastic or make things worse?

CLIENT: No, I guess not.

THERAPIST: So, it actually sounds like TV worked.

CLIENT: What do you mean?

THERAPIST: Well, you might remember what we've said about self-soothing and distraction in group—the idea that these skills can take the edge off in the short term, but the relief might not last. Also, the idea is that the skills have worked if you avoided making things worse. Do you remember that?

CLIENT: Yeah, I guess, it's just that this is so hard. The thoughts and feelings keep coming back.

THERAPIST: Right, it is incredibly hard, and I'm not surprised the thoughts and feelings keep coming back. Your brain is kind of reeling and trying to make sense of what you're going through. I wish there was something I could suggest that could lift this whole weight off you. I'm afraid the skills are really good but not that good! What kind of thoughts and feelings are you dealing with?

CLIENT: It's like, I guess guilt or something. I feel just sick that I could have ruined everything with her. It's a lot of regret. Thinking about what I should have done, what might happen, that kind of thing.

THERAPIST: I get how you might feel guilty. You did something you regret, and from what you've said, sleeping with that other woman didn't really fit your values. I would imagine, if I were you, I might also feel a little afraid that she will leave me. Does that fit?

CLIENT: Yeah, definitely worried and afraid.

THERAPIST: OK, so let's talk about how you're going to get through tonight. We're meeting in a couple of days, so we can talk then about what to do about the whole thing then. For tonight, I haven't heard you say it yet, but I'm hoping you've been able to avoid drinking. You've been doing so well with that.

CLIENT: It's true, I haven't had anything to drink. My vodka is still at my sister's house, and I really don't have anything here. I'd have to go out.

THERAPIST: Good news. Let's keep it that way. If you go out, you're not allowed to buy booze. Agreed? Remember, the number one goal of distress tolerance skills is to avoid making things worse.

CLIENT: OK, agreed.

THERAPIST: Let me ask you: Do you think you're at the point where you could experience your guilt or fear and tolerate those emotions for a while without doing anything harmful?

CLIENT: No, I really don't think so. I mean the urges to drink and stuff come up really strong, and I just can't think clearly or anything.

THERAPIST: Good to know. That's why I think we should focus on distress tolerance. Remember the distraction skills called ACCEPTS?

CLIENT: Yeah.

THERAPIST: Ok, so let's have you stack up your distress tolerance skills over the next couple of hours. When are you going to bed?

CLIENT: Oh, maybe 11:00 or so.

THERAPIST: So, we've got 3 hours. Let's come up with a little schedule. First, I'm thinking you could go back to that TV show, because it worked for a while. Second, how about doing something distracting with your brain, like those sudoku puzzles or crosswords you like in the newspaper?

CLIENT: I could do that. I would really have to concentrate, so that could be good or bad.

THERAPIST: Right, well, try it out and see what happens. Next, I suggest you have a little snack. Have you eaten yet?

CLIENT: No, I didn't really have dinner.

THERAPIST: Maybe the food should be first. Get yourself a glass of water and something that's easy to make. Then, after the puzzles, what could you do?

CLIENT: I guess I could talk to my sister. She knows Edwina really well, and she's good to talk to her. She also knows about the other woman, and she never judged me or anything.

THERAPIST: Sounds like the perfect person to talk to. Supportive but nonjudgmental. Why don't you talk with her for a while, and then wind down and get ready for bed. Remember to do all of these things mindfully. If you're ruminating or worrying the whole time, the skills aren't going to work as well. Also, if you notice they're only working for a little while, don't worry, that's how they're supposed to work. You might need to substitute or add something else. Sound workable?

CLIENT: Yeah, I can do that.

THERAPIST: OK, so remind me of what the plan is?

CLIENT: I'm going to eat a bit, watch that show, do some sudoku and crosswords from the paper, call my sister, and go to bed, right?

THERAPIST: You got it. No alcohol, and no asking your sister for the vodka, right?

CLIENT: Right.

THERAPIST: I feel good about this plan. I also think we can figure out what to do about your relationship, but table that in your mind for now. For this evening, your goal is to just get through it and not make things worse. That reminds me of one more thing. Is it possible that calling Edwina would make things worse?

CLIENT: Yeah, I think so. I kept picking up the phone earlier, but something stopped me.

THERAPIST: Probably wise. She may need some space to deal with all of this, and you might not be in the greatest shape to talk.

CLIENT: OK, I won't call her.

In this example, the clinician used a few key strategies. She checked on the skills Sam has tried so far and assessed Sam's difficulties with the skills. She then provided coaching and feedback, primarily reiterating the point that distress tolerance skills work in the short term. She validated the difficulty of what Sam is going through as well as some of his specific emotional reactions to the situation (guilt and fear). The focus turned to the idea of Sam avoiding making things worse, and the clinician got a commitment from Sam not to obtain alcohol or drink. The reader might notice that the clinician was fairly directive in stating that Sam is "not allowed" to get alcohol. This is characteristic of an irreverent therapeutic style in DBT, whereby the therapist sometimes acts omnipotent (as in this case), and at other times, acts impotent (as if she doesn't know the answer or what needs to be done) (Linehan, 1993a). Later, reflecting the fairly directive style of DBT phone coaching, the clinician also suggested that calling Edwina might make things worse and recommended against that. As time is limited, sometimes the most efficient and effective approach is to tell the client what to do or what to avoid. In addition, the clinician and Sam worked to come up with a schedule of distress tolerance activities (and support seeking by calling the sister) for the next couple of hours before bedtime. Because distress tolerance skills often work in the short term, "stacking up" the skills as the clinician suggests can be very effective. When one skill stops working, the client can move on to the next one, and so on. Finally, the clinician reminded Sam to use the skills mindfully. The astute reader might notice that some of the suggestions regarding skills coaching in Chapter 5, such as "dragging out new behavior," were not illustrated in this example. This is primarily because it would not make sense for the client to engage in some of the distress tolerance strategies while on the phone with the clinician.

Being Dialectical about Coaching in Emotion Regulation and Distress Tolerance

One key dialectic that applies here is that of acceptance versus change. As mentioned in Chapter 1 and elsewhere, DBT includes skills that focus primarily on acceptance (mindfulness skills and most of the distress tolerance skills) or change (most of the ER skills). In any situation presented by a client on the phone, it could potentially be effective to practice acceptance- or change-oriented skills or some combination of both. Any skills plan could always start with the skill of radical acceptance, as it's hard to change reality without first accepting it as it is. Balancing acceptance and change skills does not mean that a clinician should always coach clients in both types of skills during every phone coaching call. Rather, the clinician should seek to balance acceptance versus change over the longer run, across phone and other types of skills coaching.

The clinician also should use what he knows about the client and the current context to strike a useful balance of acceptance- and change-oriented skills. We once saw a client who tended to want to solve all problems that irritated her. She had tremendous difficulty keeping relationships, as she would immediately try to change anything that annoyed her. A boyfriend not texting her right back, having a cold apartment, not wearing the right clothing, or having too much of certain foods in his fridge would quickly end up on the chopping block. She similarly moved from place to place regularly due to noise, annoying landlords, poor views, and so forth. As so many aspects of life bothered her, the clinician realized that coaching in strategies to change or problem-solve life stressors could become endless. When he shifted to a focus on ways to tolerate and accept things as they are, at least temporarily, the client really began to make gains.

Summary

In summary, the majority of phone coaching calls focus on skills to help the client regulate or tolerate emotions. A model of emotions and ER can provide guidance regarding which skills to use, when, and how to respond to intense emotions during phone coaching calls. Emotions are multifaceted, generally occur in response to situations that are motivationally relevant (relevant to goals), compel various forms of action (broadly falling into the categories of approach or avoidance), and often function to communicate to others. ER has to do with how we influence the timing, experience, and expression of emotional states. ER skills in DBT are comprehensive; thus, the focus in this chapter was on two skills that can be particularly useful during phone coaching: mindfulness of current emotion and opposite action. In terms of distress tolerance, crisis survival skills can help clients tolerate strong emotions or difficult situations. These skills are practical, concrete, and ideal for the therapist to utilize during phone coaching. Crisis survival skills often work in the short term to help clients avoid engaging in behaviors that make their situation worse, and to make their emotions more bearable. These are the go-to strategies when the goal is to help the client avoid acting on impulses to engage in potentially harmful behaviors, such as drinking, using drugs, cutting, or planning suicide.

CHAPTER 7

Navigating Suicide Crisis Calls

This chapter addresses strategies and principles for navigating suicide crisis calls in the context of DBT phone coaching. While it is more ideal to help clients learn to use skills to avoid imminent suicidality, suicide crisis calls periodically occur in DBT and other treatments. In many cases, these calls are most common toward the beginning of therapy, when clients have yet to learn effective skills to manage overwhelming emotions and situations. I have observed that suicidal crises, suicide attempts, and self-injury tend to resolve for many clients within the first 4–6 months of DBT. Clients at risk of suicide, however, can display an episodic and unpredictable pattern of risk, and clinicians should be ready to address suicidal crisis at any time.

The structure and focus of suicide crisis calls generally follows guidelines from Chapter 3. Such calls ideally are (1) structured and have a beginning, middle, and end, with particular strategies often used in each segment of the call and (2) they often focus on skills to help the client regulate or tolerate emotions in the short term (described in Chapter 6). In addition, to effectively navigate such calls, it is important for the clinician to understand and use key principles to manage suicide risk, taking into account the client's unique situation. All of this needs to be done on the fly, on the phone, in a limited period of time. In this chapter, I review specific DBT suicide crisis call principles and strategies. The focus is on key facts, principles, and strategies to get started with suicide risk calls. It is important for the reader to also become familiar with the broader literature on suicide and suicide risk. As a good starting point, I highly recommend Bongar and Sullivan's (2013) book, *The Suicidal Patient: Clinical and Legal Standards of Care*.

Stylistic Strategies

In terms of therapeutic style, during suicide crisis calls, the clinician typically is active and directive, balancing the therapeutic styles of reciprocity and irreverence (Linehan, 1993a). A directive, clear, frank therapeutic style can be useful in a suicidal crisis. This is not the time to take a backseat in the therapy process or to be nondirective and simply listen empathetically. Often, it is most effective to simply tell the client what needs to be done. Marsha Linehan used to ask prospective graduate students what they would do if a client called and said she was pointing a gun at her own head. When confronted with this question, many students (and as we have found, some clinicians) waffle or say they would inquire about the problem and so forth. This is a time, however, to be directive and say something like, "Put down the gun now!" At the same time, it is crucial to convey understanding and compassion for the client's suffering. I have found that being clear and directive, in combination with structuring the phone call (see Chapter 4), can be regulating, reassuring, and anchoring to clients at sail in an emotional storm.

As mentioned in previous chapters, in DBT, the clinician often seeks to balance the therapeutic styles of reciprocity and irreverence. During suicide crisis calls, the strategic use of irreverence can help orient the client to the present moment and detach her- or himself from rigid thinking patterns. Clients who are imminently suicidal often are in a mental state characterized by high emotional arousal, rigid and repetitive thinking, and narrowed attention (i.e., cognitive deconstruction; Baumeister, 1990). Due to the often novel and unexpected nature of irreverence, it has been suggested that therapeutic irreverence prompts an orienting response (a common human response to novelty, involving increased cerebral blood flow and the preparation of neural systems for sensory analysis), essentially opening the client's attention to the present moment (Lynch, Chapman, Rosenthal, Kuo, & Linehan, 2006). When hopeless thoughts or rumination consume the client, unexpected actions or statements can temporarily help her or him focus attention on the present moment. The client is now paying attention to the clinician, rather than stuck in her or his thoughts. Irreverence in DBT commonly takes the following forms (Linehan, 1993a):

- Being matter of fact about outrageous or surprising statements or behavior: "You do know that looking up ways to kill yourself is not on our crisis plan" (likely applicable to any client).

- Commenting on factors or implications that the client does not appear to have considered. For example: "If you kill yourself, you're definitely not going to get that job" (for a client afraid of being unemployed), or "I thought you agreed not to quit therapy" (for a client stating that he will kill himself; this example comes from Linehan, 1993a).

- Using a deadpan tone of voice or demeanor.

- Making humorous, unexpected, or off-the-wall statements: "You know, the sun is overrated and bad for your skin" (in the case of an agoraphobic client who is ashamed and having suicidal thoughts because she could not get herself to go outside on a sunny day).

- Confronting the client directly in a manner that gets her or his attention: "Listen, you promised me at the beginning of therapy that you would keep yourself alive so we can improve your life. I'm going to hold you to that" (likely applicable to any client).

With irreverence, however, function is more important than form. A clinician has the flexibility to be irreverent in her or his own way. Therapeutic comments or style are irreverent if they are generally unexpected or surprising, function to get the client's attention, and spark openness to a new perspective. If irreverence does not come naturally, I recommend that clinicians practice with colleagues during mock therapy interactions or suicide crisis calls.

Flexibility, Creativity, and Therapeutic Limits

Responding to clients at imminent risk also requires flexibility and creativity. It can be useful (and indeed sometimes essential) to think outside the box, take actions that are not normally taken (e.g., agreeing to help by intervening directly in the client's environment, helping the client remove lethal means, mobilizing the client's support network, etc.), and be willing to temporarily expand the clinician's therapeutic limits to manage ongoing risk. As discussed in Chapter 8 (see also Chapman & Rosenthal, 2016), when clinicians temporarily expand their limits, it is important to (1) orient the client to the specific ways in which limits are being expanded, (2) provide a rationale for expanding limits, and (3) clarify that flexibility around limits is time-limited. An example is below.

THERAPIST: OK, I can see we are going to have to do some work to help you get unstuck from this situation. I also see that you need a little more support now than usual. Would you agree?

CLIENT: Absolutely, that's what I keep trying to tell people, but they don't seem to listen.

THERAPIST: I'm listening, and I believe you. I don't think it'll help for you to go back to the hospital. You've missed a lot of work and I'm afraid people are going to start to wonder. I don't want you to lose your job. I also don't see you staying out of the hospital and getting back on your feet without a little extra help.

CLIENT: I know, I mean, maybe I'm just better off there for a longer stay or something.

THERAPIST: You might be, and that's fine if that's what you want in your wise mind. But I think a better plan is to keep you in the game, going to work, and pulling out all the stops to use your skills. To help you do that, I'm willing to meet with you twice a week for the next 3 weeks. I also think we should have check-in calls every other day for the first week. Remember, this is a crisis, and crises pass. I'm willing to get in the boat with you for the next little while so I can help you get over the next wave.

CLIENT: I really appreciate that. I really need your help.

THERAPIST: OK, that's our plan. Keep in mind that I can only do this for 3 weeks, and then we're going to have to go back to normal. That means we both need to work hard to get you functioning, using skills, staying out of bed to stop the suicide planning, and so on. Does that sound like a deal?

CLIENT: It sounds really hard, and I can't promise anything. I really don't see any way out of this right now.

THERAPIST: Of course, I don't see how you could. You're in the middle of the storm. And, it's OK if you're not perfectly OK in 3 weeks. We'll figure out how to get over that wave if it comes. For now, though, let's get to work. The first thing I want us to do is for you to meet me early tomorrow morning with your meds so we can have the pharmacy keep them for you . . .

Core Assessment and Intervention Strategies

Core DBT assessment and intervention strategies for suicide crisis calls are similar to the general flow of strategies used to tackle any behavioral problem in DBT (see Chapter 8 of this book; see also Chapman & Rosenthal, 2016; Linehan, 1993a). Generally, the clinician (1) highlights and assesses the problem, (2) engages in collaborative problem solving, (3) obtains a commitment from the client to implement any agreed-upon solutions, and (4) troubleshoots the plan and the client's commitment. Suicide crisis calls generally involve the same strategies, with a greater emphasis on solving the most immediate problems contributing to suicide risk, generating hope and reasons for living, focusing on the client's emotional state, and planning for a recurrence of the crisis. In addition, it is important for clinicians to reflect on suicide crisis calls in a systematic and organized manner to identify any further actions that might be needed.

Briefly Assessing and Summarizing the Problem

As mentioned in Chapter 4 on the structure of phone coaching calls, one useful strategy toward the beginning of the call is to assess the events precipitating the call. In the case of suicide crisis calls, the clinician assesses the events precipitating imminent risk and the factors setting off the current crisis. Understanding these factors will help the clinician to intervene to reduce imminent risk. If, for example, the precipitant of a crisis is a breakup, the clinician might help the client avoid further interactions with the offending partner, avoid viewing her or his profile on social media, and seek alternative social support to buffer against feelings of loss or rejection. It also can be useful to briefly summarize the problem or problems setting off the crisis or imminent risk. Doing so can help the clinician and client get on the same page regarding precipitating factors.

Having clients remove themselves from prompting events for suicidal thoughts, or even from the immediate environment altogether, often is among the most effective initial strategies in reducing risk. I often have my clients immediately leave their homes and go somewhere else, where it is hard to harm themselves, such as a public library, coffee shop, friend's home, or the like. A simple change of environment often can create enough of a shift in thoughts and emotional states to help reduce risk at least temporarily.

Generating Hope

Given that hopelessness is both a robust long-term predictor of suicidal ideation and behavior (Fawcett et al., 1990; Troister, Agatha, & Holden, 2015) and a common immediate trigger for suicide-related behaviors, enhancing hope can be very helpful. Often, hope develops over the long term, when clients begin to notice that their situation can improve. During a brief crisis call, the situation may not change much, and the client may be in a cognitive state that is somewhat resistant to new information. It can, therefore, be challenging to instill hope in the context of a brief suicide crisis call. Often, I have found that preempting hope-building strategies with accurate validation of the client's suffering can help clients become more receptive to my suggestions regarding reasons for hope and reasons for living. If the client believes the clinician understands her problems, efforts to build hope are likely to seem realistic. Any of the several validation strategies used in DBT or other approaches can be helpful here, but validation level 5 (validating in terms of normative functioning or current context) (Linehan, 1993a, 1997) is particularly useful. This type of validation conveys the idea that the client's reactions are perfectly understandable given the challenges she or he is currently facing. The focus is on why the client's responses make perfect sense, rather than on why they are problematic or faulty. While it can be difficult for a clinician to find the kernel of truth to validate amid many of the extreme things a suicidal client might be saying, doing so can greatly facilitate suicide crisis calls.

Another DBT validation strategy is geared specifically toward building hope. This strategy, often referred to as *cheerleading,* involves conveying the belief that the client is capable of overcoming her or his difficulties and developing a life worth living. Cheerleading often involves encouraging and reassuring the client that things will improve in the future. The clinician also may appeal to the client's strengths, emphasizing that the client has the capabilities needed to improve her or his situation. Along these lines, the clinician may also suggest or prompt the client to recall times when she or he overcame even more difficult challenges in the past.

When using this strategy of cheerleading, it is important to be realistic. It would not be effective, for example, to try to convince a severely socially phobic individual that her dream of becoming a rock star is just around the corner. The manner and tone of cheerleading also can influence the impact of this strategy during phone coaching. I have trained many clinicians in how to effectively navigate suicide crisis calls. Part of this training involves engaging in practice calls. One of the errors that I often have observed among trainees is the tendency to be overly energetically positive when speaking to a depressed, suicidal person on the phone. While I would not usually encourage clinicians to match a client's depressive demeanor (unless this is being done strategically), overly bubbly or enthusiastic positivity can be invalidating for a client experiencing intense and unremitting suffering.

Another helpful way to instill hope is to encourage the client to engage in *opposite action* to hopeless thoughts. The idea here is much like the rationale for behavioral activation (Martell, Dimidjian, & Herman-Dunn, 2010). Often, clients need to change their mood and thoughts from the outside in, rather than from the inside out. Rather than wrestling one's brain into submission, simply taking small steps and beginning to change behavior can have a profound effect on mood and cognition.

Marita, for example, was thinking of suicide and having hopeless thoughts that her life would never change. She was in her mid-30s, living with her mother in an embattled relationship, with severe and debilitating anxiety and depression. She stated that she has always been a miserable person and can't really see any way that this situation will change in the future. She even stated that she thought that it might be best if natural selection work to weed people like her out of the gene pool (unfortunately, her prior university courses on evolution were working against her). Below is an example of how the clinician used this strategy of opposite action to combat hopelessness.

THERAPIST: You know, it occurs to me that one of the things making you suicidal right now is the idea that there is no hope that things will change, that you will be stuck living with your mom, and will never reach your goals of having a meaningful job and a family of your own. Does that sound about right?

CLIENT: Yeah, that about sums it up. I mean, I've always been so miserable, and I've never really had anything to go against that. I mean, I'm my own worst enemy. I never really learned how to be different.

THERAPIST: I know, you mentioned that your family, and your mom in particular, have been incredibly harsh and haven't really taught you to view yourself with respect. It's hard to imagine life being different from what you've been going through for so long.

CLIENT: It is really hard, I really just don't see the point of continually going through this over and over again.

THERAPIST: OK, here's what I think we need to do. I'm guessing you remember the skill of opposite action.

CLIENT: Of course, you talk about it all the time! You're obsessed with it.

THERAPIST: It is one of my favorites! In any case, you can use opposite action for thoughts . . .

CLIENT: How would I do that?

THERAPIST: Well, you sort of act as if things are hopeful. Act like you have hope even if you don't right now. Think about what you'd be doing right now if hopeful thoughts were going through your mind.

CLIENT: I don't know, I guess I'd be working on my paper that's due on Tuesday. That doesn't exactly sound like a lot of fun, though.

THERAPIST: I guess that depends on the topic, but opposite action doesn't need to be fun. I think you're on the right track, though. Why is working on your paper acting like you have hope?

CLIENT: I guess I've been working on being more independent, wanting to get out on my own. If I can finish up university and get decent marks, that might be something.

THERAPIST: Right on, I totally agree. We could think of working on your paper as one small step on the staircase out of where you are right now. Are you willing to give this idea of acting "as if" a shot?

CLIENT: Yeah, I can do that.

THERAPIST: OK, so working on your paper is a great start and I think you might need some other skills.

CLIENT: Right, I mean, I do feel pretty miserable.

THERAPIST: And with how you're feeling right now, it might also be hard to work on your paper, like difficult to concentrate and so on. Let's first think of some things you can do to shift your mood a bit. Then, we can plan for you to work on your paper, and then add other stuff to the plan, too. Sound reasonable?

CLIENT: OK.

THERAPIST: Before any of that, I want to make sure you've got suicide off the table.

CLIENT: I don't know if I can do that. I mean, I know what you're saying, but that staircase is so long. It would be so much easier just to bail.

THERAPIST: I know that sounds easier, but to have a better life, you at least have to stay on the staircase. You can take a break from time to time, but I'm asking you to stay on. And, the first thing we need to do is remove the temptation to step off. I'd like you to stay on the phone with me and lock up your pills in that box in the garage like we did before. Are you willing to do that?

In this example, the therapist targeted some of the key factors contributing to the client's suicidality, including misery and hopeless thoughts about the future. The therapist validated Marita's pain and difficulty and reminded her of the path out of misery (namely, working systematically to become more independent and get out of a toxic living situation). She coached Marita in opposite action to hopeless thoughts, and before moving on to skills to shift Marita's mood, reassessed suicide risk and asked her to take steps to remove lethal means.

Focusing on Emotions

As mentioned in other chapters, phone coaching often focuses on ways for the client to effectively regulate or tolerate emotions. Clients in a suicidal crisis often are experiencing intense, overwhelming emotional states. This can make it difficult for them to consider or use skills that involve a lot of thinking, as intense emotional states can have deleterious effects on cognition. As a result, it can often be most effective to focus not on the client's thoughts or on complicated skills requiring intact cognition, but rather on the client's current emotional state.

There are many ways to focus on emotions. One useful strategy involves the clinician directing the client's attention to her or his current emotional state. I often find it helpful to remain mindful of when the client is getting caught up in thoughts, rumination, or the content of her or his thoughts, and to gently redirect him to his current emotional experience. Remaining focused on the content of thoughts in the context of a suicidal crisis or allowing the client to ruminate out loud by venting at length about his problems often exacerbates emotional misery. The following are some helpful questions or statements that the clinician might make to help the client focus on current emotions.

- "I think we should focus on how you are feeling right now and move away from thoughts. This is because, when you're feeling as emotionally overwhelmed as you are right now, your thoughts are not likely to be too helpful. I think we need to find ways to help you get through the emotions you're feeling right now."
- "Tell me what emotions you're experiencing right now."
- "Can you describe how your emotions feel physically?"
- "Tell me a little about where in your body you feel the most intense emotion."
- "What action urges are you noticing?"
- "How intense, on a scale from zero to 10, is your emotion right now?"
- "How much, on scale from zero to 10, do you think you can tolerate how you're feeling? Zero means you can't tolerate it for another second, and 10 means you could tolerate it for the next 10 months."

Validation also can help to maintain the focus on emotions and may sometimes reduce the intensity of the client's emotional arousal. During suicide crisis calls, validation is ideally quick and accurate. The clinician must remain open to the ways in which the client's experience is valid. Recall that an important rule for validation is to validate the valid rather than the invalid. This is sometimes easier said than done, in that clients in crisis may express a number of extreme opinions, thoughts, judgments, and emotions. The clinician's challenge is to identify the kernel of truth in what the client is experiencing. Often, that kernel of truth may be the fact that it is incredibly difficult to be skillful and to keep going in the middle of an emotional storm. Recall from Chapter 6 that strong emotions often function to communicate. In the case of a suicide crisis, the client's intense emotions may function to communicate her intense pain. If this message seems to get through, that pain may diminish to a level at which the client can use effective skills.

Solving the Current Problem

Often the best way to navigate a suicide crisis is to solve the immediate problem precipitating the crisis. I find it helpful to let clients know that

I think of suicide as one potential solution to a problem. The problem might be emotional pain, physical pain, persistent and stressful life circumstances, relationship turmoil, problems in functioning, and so forth. I tell clients that, although suicide seems like a solution to these problems and suicidal thoughts can be somewhat comforting, there are likely many other possible solutions. When clients become focused on suicide as the way to solve a problem, they are unlikely to step back, view the problem from a broader perspective, and entertain alternative solutions. The clinician should encourage the mindset that when suicidal thoughts occur, this means there is a problem to solve. The first step in solving that problem is to identify it. I often recommend that clients use suicidal thoughts as a signal to ask themselves the question, "What problem am I trying to solve?" On the phone, I find it helpful to remind clients of this way of thinking about suicide and ask them what problem they are trying to solve. I also often ask, "All things considered, would you rather be dead or would you rather solve this problem (e.g., be in less emotional pain, have fewer problems in your relationship, and so forth)?" The vast majority of my clients have said that they would rather solve the problem; they just don't know how to do it and are so distraught that it seems impossible to do anything about the problem. The clinician, therefore, must be an excellent problem-solver. To do this, it is helpful to know some of the basic steps for problem solving (also outlined in the emotion regulation section of Linehan, 2015): (1) describe the problem; (2) check the facts; (3) describe the problem again (if the initial description was not clear, objective, or specific enough); (4) brainstorm possible solutions; (5) evaluate a couple of promising solutions, often by entertaining pros and cons; (6) implement the solution(s); and (7) evaluate the outcomes. In a brief phone coaching call, it can be hard to fit in all of these steps. The clinician must quickly assess the most pressing problem associated with the client's suicide risk and help the client identify his goals and come up with some concrete solutions that are easy to implement. It can be helpful to remind clients of the four options to solve any problem (described in Linehan, 2015): (1) solve the problem, involving fixing or changing the situation; (2) change one's emotional reaction to the problem, involving cognitive (e.g., reappraisal) or behavioral (e.g., opposite action) strategies to modulate emotions; (3) accept or tolerate the problem, involving radical acceptance or other distress tolerance strategies (Linehan, 2015); or (4) stay miserable, which does not require any particular skill or therapeutic assistance. I often have clients memorize these four options to solve problems so that when crises hit, they are able to quickly determine which skills to use.

Many problems setting off suicidality are not solvable in a short phone call. The client's problems in relationships, for example, might be complex and require several sessions to understand. When this is the case, I often remind the client that while we will not be able to solve these problems in a short phone call, we will work on them together in our therapy sessions. I also find it useful to convey hope that, together, we will find a way to work effectively on whatever problems they are facing. During the phone call, I try to boil things down to the emotions the client is having the most difficult time tolerating and skills she can use to tolerate or regulate these emotions. It can also be helpful to identify ways that the client might make the situation worse and use problem-solving strategies to help the client take a different approach. If the client, for example, is suicidal because she is distraught after a breakup, the therapist might encourage her to avoid checking her ex-boyfriend's social media posts, calling him to try to get him back, or spending time with common friends. If the client is sad and lonely and has urges to engage in unsafe sexual encounters, the therapist might coach him on alternative ways to feel connected to others.

Getting a Commitment to a Plan

It is standard practice in DBT for the clinician to use motivational and commitment strategies to secure a commitment to any solutions that have been generated. The principle is that people are more likely to follow through on changes in behavior if they make a public commitment to do so. In the context of crisis calls, it can be crucial to obtain a commitment from the client to implement a plan to reduce suicide risk. If the client has not agreed to undertake the plan, is very difficult to know whether the client will take any steps to reduce his or her risk.

There are several strategies in DBT to encourage the client to commit to behavior change (Linehan, 1993a). Many of the strategies overlap considerably with those used in motivational interviewing (see Miller & Rollnick, 2012). Although the clinician may use the same strategies during a suicide crisis call as he or she would employ during an individual therapy session, the stakes are higher during suicide crisis calls. The clinician, therefore, is likely to be more directive during suicide crisis calls compared with regular phone coaching calls or individual therapy sessions. During a 10-minute call in which the client is imminently suicidal, the clinician who confines her- or himself solely to using reflective listening, empathy, and rolling with resistance will probably have difficulty helping the client take action to reduce risk. A directive approach might involve the clinician stating that she or he is going to need the client to commit to the plan, explicitly conveying the importance of committing to the plan, selling commitment by emphasizing the benefits of following through with the plan, among other strategies. Perhaps more so than at any other time, the clinician is likely to simply tell the client what to do during suicide crisis calls.

Below is a continuation of the example of Marita above, after she has gone to lock up the pills in the garage.

THERAPIST: Great, I'm glad we've gotten the pills out of the way for now. I know that was a bit of a leap of faith on your part . . . [*They subsequently discuss distress tolerance skills Marita can use before working on her paper.*]

THERAPIST: Here's what I'd like you to do. As agreed, you're going to try the TIP skills by going for a short run, and then take a warm bath when you get back. After you're refreshed, you'll work on your paper for maybe an hour or so, and then reward yourself by watching something you really like—something really engaging that grabs your attention. Are we agreed?

CLIENT: Yeah, I guess I can try to do that.

THERAPIST: You know I never let a "try" pass me by. What do you mean by "try"?

CLIENT: I'll do the run and the bath, and then work on my paper, OK?

THERAPIST: OK, but what about the TV and stuff afterward?

CLIENT: I can do that, but I don't know how I'm going to feel.

THERAPIST: I'm asking you to jump in mindfully with both feet and just do the plan regardless of how you feel. I know this is hard, but you did agree to pull out all the stops to keep yourself alive during therapy, remember?

CLIENT: Yeah, I remember.

THERAPIST: So, I'm asking you to keep that commitment and do what we've agreed on this evening. There's always another day to kill yourself if you really want to. I can't really stop you. I just don't want that day to be today.

CLIENT: I can agree it won't be today.

THERAPIST: Good, and I also think we need more time than a couple of days to shape up your life. Would you agree?

CLIENT: Yeah.

THERAPIST: So, I'd like you to give me time here. I'd love it if you could jump in and reaffirm your commitment to give me time to help you. That means no suicide while you're working with me. You need to be alive for me to help you.

CLIENT: I have to think about that. I don't know why I agreed to that in the first place.

THERAPIST: It's hard to see right now, and I think this could be a longer conversation than we can have right now. Let's do this: You agree to do the plan we've discussed, keep the pills in the garage, and no hurting yourself or trying to kill yourself at least until we meet. Then, we can talk more long term. Sound OK? You've gotten through a hellish past couple of weeks, so I'm confident you can do this.

CLIENT: Yeah, I can definitely do that.

THERAPIST: Great, and we're going to talk about the long term on Tuesday. We can't just go day to day or week to week, and I'm sure you know that . . .

Troubleshooting

Troubleshooting involves anticipating potential obstacles to the implementation or effectiveness of the plan to reduce suicide risk. Troubleshooting during phone coaching should be quick and efficient. It can be effective for the clinician to use what she or he knows about the client to anticipate and state possible obstacles. A client with deficits in assertiveness skills, for example, might agree to a plan that he does not intend to implement. If the clinician knows this, she or he might say something like, "Is there any chance that you might just be agreeing to all of this, but that, when we get off the phone, you might not actually do it?"

The clinician may also suggest common obstacles that might prevent any of us from putting a plan into action. Within the DBT skills training manual, Linehan (2015) has outlined a new strategy, called the *missing links analysis*. This strategy most commonly is used in group skills training to understand why clients may not have done their homework and what factors need to be addressed to make homework more successful next time around. For the reader who is familiar with DBT, a missing links analysis is much like an abbreviated chain analysis. Within a missing links analysis, the clinician suggests a few common factors that often impede homework compliance, including (1) lack of understanding of the assignment, (2) lack of willingness to do the assignment, (3) failure to remember to do the assignment, and (4) other possible factors. A missing links analysis, however, can be used as a guiding framework for troubleshooting suicide risk or other behavioral plans. Below, I have modified the questions typically used in a missing links analysis. These questions can help facilitate troubleshooting during suicide crisis calls:

- "Do you know what you need to do? Do you understand the plan? If not, what questions do you have?"
- "Are you willing to put our plan into action? If not, what's getting in the way of your willingness to use our plan?"
- "Do you think you will remember to do our plan? If not, what might help you remember?"
- "Can you think of any other obstacles that might prevent our plan from working, or prevent you from doing it?"

Anticipating That the Crisis May Recur

Another important step in suicide crisis calls is to anticipate and plan for the possible return or recurrence of the crisis. The clinician does not assume that, following the call, the client's risk is nonexistent. Indeed, crises come and go, and complex clients may often demonstrate the pattern that Linehan (1993a) has labeled "unrelenting crisis." The client, for example, might get off the phone, implement distress tolerance skills, remove potentially lethal means, and so on, only to get a phone call from her ex-boyfriend that precipitates another suicidal crisis. At other times, the crisis may seem to have passed, but the client's emotional pain may have waned temporarily before another wave rushes in. Therefore, it is effective (and often crucial) to remain vigilant and aware that the crisis may not pass or may recur.

Knowing that the crisis may recur, the clinician often maintains some form of contact with the client. The clinician might, for example, use one or more of the following strategies:

- Schedule a check-in call for later on.
- Have the client call her or him after implementing some aspect of the plan, such as removing lethal means or traveling to a friend or relative's home.
- Schedule an in-person session for earlier in the week than usual.
- Maintain contact with supports or loved ones (if desirable, and in keeping with the principles of DBT case management; see Linehan, 1993).
- Encourage the client to call back if she or he needs more help or to report on how effective the skills have been.
- Set up a time and place to meet if in-person assistance is critical.

In DBT, this is what is often called "staying close in a crisis." Staying close in a crisis has a few key benefits: (1) helping the clinician quickly observe any deterioration or increases in risk, (2) facilitating quick and efficient crisis planning or modifications to existing plans, and (3) helping the client feel supported and connected during a difficult time. Although these strategies may be demanding for the clinician, ideally the clinician and client will collaborate to reduce suicidal crises over time. If the clinician is concerned about burnout related to suicidal crises, she or he should speak to the client about this concern and seek support and consultation from colleagues (please see section below).

There are a couple of key principles to keep in mind when staying close in a crisis. First, the clinician should maintain awareness of the possible contingencies maintaining suicidality. Increased therapeutic attention and support sometimes reinforce suicidal crises. As a result, I often recommend against the clinician telling the client that she or he should call if suicidal thoughts or urges become more intense, if the client is having more difficulty, and so on. Telling a client that she or he should call if skills are not working, if she is suicidal, or if a crisis occurs or recurs risks creating a contingency whereby therapeutic support differentially reinforces crisis behavior and suicidality. When this is the contingency, the client also might come to believe that she must be in dire straits (or be suicidal) in order to get extra help and support. As a result, I tend to prefer noncontingent, scheduled check-in calls. For example, I recently spoke with a client who was having difficulty resisting self-harm urges. We devised a schedule of distress tolerance activities for her to engage in during the evening, but I remained concerned that the crisis would persist; thus, I told the client I would call back in 3 hours to check in and answer any questions she might have about the skills she was trying. I briefly oriented the client to the subsequent call, emphasizing that the focus should be on skills coaching. This strategy ensures that help is not contingent on suicidality and that the client is aware that any calls will focus on skills coaching.

A second important principle to keep in mind is that, in DBT crisis calls, the clinician usually uses conservative strategies until they stop working and then entertains less conservative strategies. Conservative strategies include those that are least restrictive, involve minimal environmental interventions, and encourage the client to take charge of reducing her or his risk. Less conservative strategies are more restrictive and often involve environmental interventions or unconventional approaches. An example of a conservative approach is to conduct a suicide crisis call as described in this chapter, help the client solve the immediate problem, secure a commitment to lower risk and use skills, troubleshoot, and so on. If the client, for example, remains at high risk and is unwilling to commit to a plan to reduce risk, a less conservative approach would be to involve others in the client's support network in reducing risk, encourage the client to go to the hospital (or facilitating this), contact the police, meet the client to retrieve medications and prevent an overdose, take the client to the emergency room, and so forth. The basic rule is to use less conservative strategies only if conservative strategies have failed. In DBT, the threshold is high for recommending hospitalization or breaching confidentiality to ensure safety, although these options are always available in the event of imminent suicide risk. Below is a list of common strategies, from least to most conservative.

- Assessing risk, coaching the client in skills to reduce risk, securing a commitment, and troubleshooting.
- Remaining more available than usual in a crisis for additional phone coaching.
- Remaining more available than usual for extra in-person meetings.

- Coaching the client to enlist natural supports in reducing risk.
- Helping the client contact natural supports to reduce risk.
- Contacting the client's natural supports on her or his behalf.
- Urging the client to go to the hospital, call the ambulance, or call the police.
- Taking the client to the hospital, calling an ambulance, or calling the police.

Reevaluating, Documenting, and Consulting as Needed

Even if suicide risk is addressed thoroughly by using all of the strategies mentioned in this chapter, it is still important to reflect and reevaluate. Consistent with dialectical principles, in DBT phone coaching it is useful to consider what might be missing from any intervention or plan. A seemingly watertight plan may have a leak somewhere. The client may, for example, have committed to avoiding suicidal behavior, using distress tolerance skills, seeking support from others, removing potentially lethal medications, and checking in later on. The clinician may end the call feeling comfortable about the client's suicide risk, only to hear later that the client has been hospitalized after an attempt to run into traffic. It is easy to miss the myriad destabilizing factors influencing the client's ongoing suicide risk. The client might still attempt suicide following an unexpected prompting event, find the skills discussed to be ineffective, fail to use the skills, or have a suicide plan of which the clinician is unaware. Therefore, rather than getting off the phone reassured that the client will be safe, it is helpful for the clinician to reflect on the call and consider anything that might have been missed.

The Linehan Risk Assessment and Management Protocol

One way to reflect and reevaluate is to use a structured suicide risk documentation method or protocol. One such protocol is the Linehan Risk Assessment and Management Protocol (LRAMP; Linehan, 2014). The LRAMP is freely available at *http://blogs.uw.edu/brtc/files/2014/01/SSN-LRAMP-updated-9-19_2013.pdf,* and an online version requiring a subscription is available at *www.behavioraltech.org.* The LRAMP is both a protocol and a documentation method. The LRAMP has several sections corresponding to important domains to consider and document:

- **Section 1 (reason for completing)** inquires about the reasons the clinician is completing the LRAMP. Some of these may include increased suicidal ideation, behavior, threats, or other signs of increased risk.

- **Section 2 (specific incident or behavior)** involves describing the specific situation prompting the completion of the LRAMP. This might, for example, be a brief description of the suicidal crisis call.

- **Section 3 (structured formal assessment of suicide risk)** inquires as to whether a structured, formal assessment of suicide risk was completed and provides check boxes for various reasons as to why such assessment might not have been completed. My personal favorite check box is "forgot."

- **Section 4 (imminent risk factors)** includes a list of imminent risk factors to consider for this particular client.

- **Similarly Section 5 (suicide protective factors)** includes a list of common protective factors.

- **Section 6 (treatment actions)** includes a variety of check boxes having to do with different treatment actions that may or may not have been conducted. Such treatment actions may include a behavioral or chain analysis, crisis intervention strategies, commitment, troubleshooting, and other strategies discussed in this chapter.

- **Section 7 (final disposition)** includes the clinician's final determination of the client's current risk. When risk is rated as low, the check boxes require the clinician to indicate why, such as suicidal ideation/intent have reduced, there is a crisis plan in place, protective factors outweigh risk factors, and so on. Section 7 also includes a plan for follow-up/reevaluation of risk.

Methods such as the LRAMP encouraged the clinician to think through her or his decisions regarding suicide risk and to consider as much information as possible. I have often completed the LRAMP and then realized that I may have missed something potentially important and should consult with a colleague and follow-up with the client. This also has happened several times with my supervisees. A student was completing an LRAMP several months ago and realized that, while the client agreed to a safety plan, she had not discussed specific skills the client could use to reduce risk, and they had not troubleshot factors that might increase the client's risk (in this case, further spousal conflict).

The student called me, and after reviewing what she had done, I urged her to call the client back. It was fortunate that she did, as there had just been a blowup with the spouse, the client was distraught, and she had begun to look for ways to harm herself. Whether the clinician is using the LRAMP or some other method, reviewing and documenting suicide crisis calls promptly (and possibly discussing them with a colleague) can alert her or him to any need for further action.

Consultation

It also can be useful to consistently consult with a colleague or group of colleagues regarding suicide crisis calls. Colleagues can help identify factors that the clinician might have missed or forgotten to raise or plan for. While immediate consultation following a suicide crisis call is not always possible, I would highly recommend that clinicians consult on a regular basis with colleagues if they regularly receive suicide crisis calls. In the context of a DBT program, this consultation generally occurs through the DBT consultation team (discussed in Chapter 2), which meets weekly. Two specific categories of standing DBT consultation team agenda items pertain to suicide crisis calls: imminent risk and life-threatening behaviors. If I have conducted a suicide crisis call and believe the client is at ongoing imminent risk, I put that client on the agenda under the category of imminent risk. Typically, that category is the first to be discussed in the meeting. If the risk appears to have passed, but the client was at moderate-to-high suicide risk during the crisis call, I would put her or him on the agenda for life-threatening behavior. In DBT consultation teams, the clinician is expected to let the team know what she wants or needs from the team. Generally, in many DBT teams, the clinician's needs generally fall within one of four different categories:

- **Help with assessment**. In this case, the clinician needs help better understanding a problem situation or behavior. In the case of suicide crisis calls, the clinician might need to better understand factors contributing to suicide risk, areas that were missed, or areas that require further assessment.

- **Help with problem solving**. This involves seeking consultation regarding ways to effectively intervene to reduce suicide risk, or to solve the longer-term problems contributing to suicidality (e.g., depression, chronic misery, problems in the client's living situation). I have found this to be the most commonly expressed need of clinicians when suicide crisis calls have recently occurred. The team's function here is to help the clinician devise effective interventions to not only manage risk but to solve the problems in living that contribute to ongoing risk. In DBT, the goal is to develop a life worth living, rather than to keep the client on life support.

• **Assistance in increasing empathy for the client**. In the context of suicide crisis calls, this category is often used when the clinician begins to notice signs of burnout and compassion fatigue. Irritability and frustration with the client, reductions in willingness to help the client, the experience of dreading the client's call, and so on, often indicate that suicide crisis calls present a risk of burnout. The client may be calling too often, engaging in aversive behavior on the phone, or experiencing chronic, unremitting suicide risk that the clinician finds overwhelming. In these cases, the team's function is often to help shore up the clinician's motivation to continue to help and build empathy for the client.

• **Support and validation**. At times, clinicians working with imminently suicidal clients simply need support and validation from others who know what it's like to engage in this kind of work. Although team members may notice that the clinician also needs help with assessment or problem solving (and may provide such help), it is helpful to place priority on the clinician's need for support and validation.

Most commonly, if I have had a suicide crisis call that I wish to speak with the team about, I often place it in the category of assessment or problem solving. This way, the team knows I need help further assessing the situation and the client's potential ongoing suicide risk, or additional ways to help the client lower her or his risk. At times, if I am receiving repeated suicide risk calls that threatened to burn me out in the long run, I may raise this issue during the team meeting (under the category of therapy-interfering behavior), seeking support, validation, or problem-solving suggestions on how to prevent burnout.

For those clinicians who are not currently involved with a DBT team, it can be useful to have a consistent consultation network and to structure consultation in a way that is similar to the structure of the DBT team. When consulting with a colleague individually in an ad-hoc manner, the clinician might consider what she or he needs from that colleague and state this upfront. I also recommend that the clinician ask a colleague to point out if she or he has missed anything. Some colleagues can be reluctant to give directive or critical feedback. To get around this potential problem, I recommend that clinicians convey the message that even though they have done their best, they have probably missed something, and they would welcome any critical feedback or suggestions on anything they might have missed. The clinician also must be willing to be vulnerable, upfront, and clear about her or his worries or concerns.

Being Dialectical about Suicide Crisis Calls

Suicide has many inherent dialectics. A common dialectic is the tension between the clinician's values and her or his professional obligations. Some clinicians value free will and autonomy and believe clients should have the right to die. This value is sometimes at odds with professional obligations to take steps to reduce the chances that a client or specific other(s) will come to harm. I once had a client who made me think about this dialectic. He suffered from treatment-resistant depression; had a prolonged history of invalidation, trauma, and abuse; was socially isolated; and suffered from serious functional impairments. We worked together for a long time, and he made minimal progress. Although he became somewhat more active and started working toward personal (becoming independent and leaving his parents' home) and occupational (working toward completion of graduate program) goals, his prolonged episodes of depression always returned and were nonresponsive to medication and only minimally responsive to therapy. He barely slept for more than 3 or 4 hours per night, spent much of his time in his home, had a toxic relationship with his family, and had persistent, intractable shame about treatment that often road-blocked therapy and the therapy relationship. He was miserable, had been so for many years, and had almost convinced me that he was likely to continue to be miserable for the foreseeable future. One day, he asked me if I would help him die if things continued this way. He asked why I think his situation is so different from someone with a terminal physical illness. Although I gave him the expected, professional answer focusing on my obligations, this client challenged me to think about my values.

I believe clinicians who work with suicidal clients should ask themselves difficult questions, examine their beliefs, and engage with this possible dialectic. Engaging with the dialectic does not mean that you have to solve it or come up with a synthesis right away. There often is no easy synthesis when it comes to suicide. When I do trainings in DBT and on the assessment and treatment of suicidal behavior, I often ask people to consider a few key questions (some of these questions also are asked in the context of intensive DBT training offered through Behavioral Tech, LLC):

- "What are your beliefs about death?"
- "What are your values or beliefs about whether people have the right to commit suicide?"
- "What are your obligations in working with an imminently suicidal client?"
- "How do these obligations fit with your values?"
- "If your values and obligations are in polarity, what is a possible synthesis?"

Another common dialectic is between the following two ideas: (1) clients need to take suicide off the table in order to build a life worth living, and (2) to get suicide off the table, it is often necessary to build a life worth living. In the midst of intense, unrelenting misery, it is hard to imagine taking suicide off the table without the promise of some relief; thus, the clinician's job is to help the client solve the problems contributing to suicidality while simultaneously helping the client to keep suicide off the table. Moving completely to one pole or the other is ineffective and dangerous. Therapy focusing entirely on suicide and suicide risk devolves into crisis management, and treatment focused entirely on solving the misery of the client's life (without adequately managing suicide risk) can put the client's life at risk. While phone coaching can help solve problems contributing to misery in the short run, suicide crisis calls inevitably must focus on the immediate reduction of suicide risk. I try to think of each phone coaching call, in conjunction with ongoing work on suicidality in individual DBT, as a sculptor's chipping off a piece of stone. Each call might not seem to make a tremendous difference, but over time, as the client continues to survive crises and use skills effectively, the statue begins to emerge.

Summary

In summary, suicide crisis calls involve many of the same structural and therapeutic strategies used in other types of phone coaching calls. It is important to structure suicide crisis calls and to use the principles of targeting to give suicidal crises high priority. Stylistically, it can be useful to balance the therapeutic styles of irreverence and reciprocity. Irreverence can help the client shift focus and view her or his situation from a different perspective, and warm engagement and validation can help regulate the client's emotions. It can be effective to focus on emotions, use validation strategies, and emphasize actions the client can take in the here and now. Understanding the prompting events for the crisis can directly suggest ways to reduce risk in the short term (e.g., by having the client reduce contact with prompting events). Other core strategies include assessment, problem solving, commitment, and troubleshooting. The clinician also should consider whether the crisis situation necessitates some flexibility in therapeutic limits. In addition, it is important to anticipate the possible reemergence of the crisis, to reflect on decisions, and to seek help and consultation as needed.

CHAPTER 8

Principles and Strategies to Address Challenges and Observe Limits

Although phone coaching often enhances therapy and the therapy relationship, and the vast majority of clients use phone coaching constructively, challenges periodically arise. Clients may call more frequently or wish to talk at length, call repeatedly in crisis, seek help other than skills coaching (e.g., for therapy on the phone, to alleviate loneliness), text or e-mail prodigiously and expect an immediate response, become angry and critical, refuse to use or discuss skills, and much more. Indeed, I often tell clinicians that they are bound to encounter a small number of clients (perhaps two or three) who will make them wish they never got involved in phone coaching in the first place. Moreover, clinicians themselves also sometimes interfere with the effective use of phone coaching, perhaps most commonly by allowing their limits to be stretched to the point of burnout, remaining on the phone for too long, trying to do therapy on the phone, failing to return calls, becoming frustrated with clients on the phone (or over electronic communication methods), among several other examples. This chapter focuses on effective, compassionate approaches to therapy-interfering behaviors (TIBs) arising in the context of phone coaching, with a particular focus on strategies to observe limits.

Principles for Addressing Therapy-Interfering Behavior

As defined by Chapman and Rosenthal (2016) and elsewhere (Farmer & Chapman, 2016; Linehan, 1993a), TIB is any behavior on the part of the client or clinician that (1) makes it difficult to implement treatment, (2) hampers the client's progress, or (3) makes it difficult to work effectively with the client. With this definition in mind, a few key principles and steps can help the clinician effectively manage TIB arising in the context of phone coaching.

Define and Conceptualize Client and Clinician TIB Functionally

In DBT, TIB is defined functionally by its effect on therapy or the therapy relationship, not topographically in terms of the specific form of the behavior. A client yelling at the clinician on the phone, for example, would be engaging in TIB only if his or her yelling hampers skills coaching, the client's progress, or the therapy relationship (perhaps by upsetting the clinician, eliciting fear, or pushing the clinician's limits). Complaints about treatment or threats to quit may be TIB, making it hard to proceed with phone coaching and hampering productive discussions about skills. Such behaviors, however, also present opportunities to assess and understand the client's experiences, her or his goals, and whether progress is occurring. In other cases, some behaviors are TIB by default, such as when a client hangs up on the clinician, or when the clinician fails to return a client call. In either of these cases, phone coaching is cut short or can't occur.

When conceptualizing TIB, it is also useful to consider the functional properties of the behavior. While the overt topography of TIB often commands attention when, for example, a client has called or texted for the 40th time that week, effectively addressing TIB often requires a precise understanding of the function or utility of the behavior. In this regard, it is useful to consider the following key factors.

- The context in which the TIB occurs
- The antecedents to TIB, both in terms of external events and internal events (the client's thoughts, emotions, expectations, etc.)

- The specific form, frequency, duration, and intensity of the TIB
- The consequences, possibly including reinforcers that might maintain TIB

Understanding TIB within this *functional analysis* framework will help the clinician generate hypotheses to test and highlight potentially helpful solutions. Consistent with this functional view is the idea that the clinician's thoughts about why the client is engaging in the behavior are simply hypotheses to be tested. As with any clinically relevant behavior, clinicians should avoid becoming attached to their hypotheses and to be willing to discard them in the face of refuting evidence.

This functional view of TIB also applies to the clinician. It is easy for clinicians to slip into TIB during phone coaching. Some examples might be allowing phone calls to go on for too long, moving out of role (doing individual therapy instead of skills coaching on the phone), becoming judgmental of the client, failing to return calls, returning calls too soon, breaking commitments to the client (e.g., that she or he will be available or will call at a certain time), and so on. The challenge for the clinician is to notice, early in the process, when he or she is engaging in TIB, and to reflect on the context, antecedents, and functions of such TIB. In DBT and other team-based approaches, the clinician need not do all this work alone. On our team, for example, we expect clinicians to raise their own possible TIB each week so that the team can help them understand and overcome it. Clinicians also are expected to observe signs of impending burnout and to seek help and support well before burnout strikes. To make this a routine part of our team meetings, we ask clinicians to provide burnout ratings (0 = not burned out at all to 10 = completely burned out and unable to go on) before the meeting starts.

Maintain a Mindful, Nonjudgmental Stance

Another useful principle is to maintain a mindful, nonjudgmental stance regarding TIB. Mindful awareness of the effect of the client's behavior on therapy or the therapy relationship is required to effectively observe limits, as described later in this chapter. Furthermore, a nonjudgmental stance will help the clinician avoid unnecessary suffering and counter-therapeutic behavior. Clinicians might be inclined, for example, to judge frequent or lengthy calls as "neediness" or an indication of the client's interpersonal pathology. It also is easy to judge clients who do not cooperate with problem solving or suggestions regarding skills as "resistant," "hostile," or unmotivated to change. These judgments, however, are never helpful.

As we teach clients in DBT, judgments often come with an unfortunate emotional cost. When a clinician judges a client as hostile or needy, for example, clinician frustration or even contempt for the client are likely to follow. Furthermore, much like a stereotype, the judgmental label may narrow the clinician's attention and information processing, such that information consistent with the judgment is processed more readily, and inconsistent information is neglected or discounted. Aside from increased stress and distorted information processing, this process can contribute to compassion fatigue and ineffective behaviors. Indeed, the early signs of impending burnout may include increased frequency of negative judgments about a client or a client's behaviors (as illustrated in Dan's Story in Box 8.1). Such judgments both result from negative reactions to the client's behavior (e.g., frustration, annoyance, sadness) and amplify these reactions.

There are many ways for clinicians to practice nonjudging. The most important first step is to become aware of judgments when they are occurring. To do this, I recommend that clinicians familiarize themselves with the mindfulness skill of *nonjudging* as described in the *DBT Skills Training Manual, 2nd Edition* (Linehan, 2015). Judgments involve placing people, events, behaviors, emotions, or thoughts into evaluative categories, such as "good," "bad," "right," "wrong," "should," "shouldn't," or other variants of these categories. When a clinician mindfully recognizes judgmental thoughts, he or she can practice letting go of the judgments and attending to the facts at hand or actively replacing the judgments with more accurate statements of fact. Regarding the latter, I have often told clients and clinicians that the DBT mindfulness skill of *describe* (Linehan, 1993b, 2015) is the antidote to judging. To describe a client's "needy" behavior, the clinician might state, "She calls me twice per day and several times over the weekend. She often calls when she's lonely, sad, and needs social support." Turning judgments into descriptions of specific facts reduces emotional suffering and usually provides a clearer path forward. It's difficult to treat "neediness" as a general trait, but it is possible to target the client's loneliness, sadness, need for social support, and frequent calls.

BOX 8.1. Overcoming Judgments: Dan's Story

One clinician, Dan, for example, overextended himself and was readily available for multiple phone calls, texts, and e-mails. He did this out of concern for the client, who was repeatedly in suicidal crisis, being victimized physically and sexually, and having difficulty with housing. Dan initially extended his limits in hopes that the crises would pass, and that the phone coaching (and e-mails, texts, etc.) would normalize to a more manageable level. Dan quickly realized, however, that the client was experiencing "unrelenting crises" (Linehan, 1993a). The crises were unlikely to pass anytime soon, and the clinician was overwhelmed and became resentful about the client's incursion on his personal time. He began to judge the client as overly needy, manipulative, and inconsiderate. He tried to observe limits around phone coaching, but discussions often devolved quickly. The therapist became sharp with the client, the client felt hurt and withdrew, and tried to call less often for a brief period, but the changes were fleeting, and as this cycle continued, the therapy relationship began to erode. After consulting with his team, Dan realized that, to effectively address this issue, he had to start by practicing nonjudging, use strategies to regulate his own emotions, and seek ways to reinvigorate his empathy for the client. He also had to observe and set firm and consistent limits and avoid deviating in order to prevent the intermittent reinforcement of the behaviors that were burning him out.

Approach TIB as a Valuable Therapeutic Opportunity

Viewing TIB as a valuable opportunity can help the client and clinician learn and grow from challenges occurring during phone coaching. TIB often presents opportunities that would not otherwise arise. I saw a client, for example, who often called me when she was lonely and sad. We worked on skills to tolerate loneliness and sadness, and she often felt better toward the end of our calls. I felt good about helping her, and she felt good about calling. Talking on the phone was reinforcing for both of us (negatively reinforcing for the client and positively reinforcing for me). The problem, however, was that she started calling so frequently that I could not keep up the level of support she needed. Furthermore, she often called before trying other skills for manage sadness or loneliness. Her go-to skill had become calling me and asking for help. When we discussed this issue, she disclosed that this pattern had arisen in other relationships: she often sought a degree of support that others were unable to sustain, and this led to people avoiding her, amplifying her loneliness and sadness. We had stumbled into an important therapy target that could have broad effects on the quality of her relationships. Indeed, TIB occurring in the therapy relationship often presents an important opportunity precisely because it echoes the challenges the client faces in other spheres of life (Chapman & Rosenthal, 2016).

Use a Dialectical and Systemic Approach

While addressing TIB around phone coaching, put dialectical theory into action. Dialectical theory reminds the clinician that therapy is a system and a relationship. If a client is calling too frequently, this might be seen as the client's problem. Dialectical theory, however, reminds us that there are always at least two valid sides to every story. It's likely, for example, that the clinician's behaviors reinforce frequent calling in some way, as in the example described just above. Dialectical theory reminds the clinician to think systemically about TIB, considering the role of the client, the clinician, and the context of the therapy relationship.

A dialectical approach also helps the clinician consider aspects of the client's perspective that are understandable, wise, or valid. If the client, for example, is calling 40 times per week, it may seem as if the client's perspective is completely invalid. Who wants to take 40 calls per week? Why would anyone think it's reasonable to call their therapist (or anyone for that matter) 40 times per week? Clearly, this behavior is dysfunctional. The challenge, though, is to search for the wisdom or validity in the client's perspective or behavior. Perhaps the client genuinely needs a lot of social support or help, does not know how to manage or tolerate loneliness, finds the calls incredibly reinforcing, or is actually being helped by all of this between-session contact. These are just hypotheses. To discover the validity in the client's perspective, the clinician must assess the problem from a vantage point that is open to the wisdom in the client's point of view.

As another example, a client may call and then refuse to talk about skills, denigrate the clinician and the therapy, and vent at length about his or her problems. What could be valid about the client's position in this case? Some hypotheses and the potential solutions stemming from them are as follows. There are, of course, many other possibilities. I include these as examples of how searching for the wisdom or truth in the client's behavior or experiences can pave the way for effective intervention strategies.

- *The client may experience the clinician's suggestions regarding skills to be invalidating.* Distraction and self-soothing skills, for example, might seem like simple solutions to the client's complex and pervasive suffering. It may be effective for the clinician to step back and accurately validate the client's emotional experiences, including the experience of being offered what seem to be overly simplistic solutions. The clinician also might explain that, while the solution seems simple, it is the best they can do in a short call. Over the long run, therapy can more extensively address and hopefully solve the problems contributing to the client's suffering.

- *The client might not understand the skills and feel frustrated that the clinician keeps suggesting them.* In this case, the clinician might validate the difficulty of being asked to do things she or he does not understand and help the client to better understand the skills.

- *The client might not have been adequately oriented to the goals and structure of phone coaching.* As a result, it is frustrating to be offered skills when he or she was simply calling for support. The client also may be socially isolated and have limited opportunities to talk about stressful events in daily life (thus, the venting). Some solutions to these problems could include (1) reorienting the client to the goals, structure, and expectations of phone coaching; (2) helping the client establish new social connections; (3) discussing the potentially negative effects of prolonged "venting" and suggesting alternative ways to express concerns or manage distress.

Steps for Managing TIP

Several key steps can help clinicians effectively manage TIB in the context of standard practice generally and phone coaching specifically. These steps also appear elsewhere (Farmer & Chapman, 2016; Linehan, 1993a) and are elaborated and applied to a variety of TIBs from a DBT perspective in Chapman and Rosenthal (2016). These steps are listed and briefly defined in Table 8.1. It is not always necessary to complete every step or to complete them in this exact order. Also, due to space

TABLE 8.1. Steps for Addressing Therapy-Interfering Behavior

Identify the behavior as therapy interfering.

The clinician attends to the client's (or clinician's own) behavior, observes and describes it without judgments or assumptions, and considers the effects of the behavior on the implementation or effectiveness of therapy or on the therapy relationship. The clinician also considers the treatment hierarchy in DBT and determines how to prioritize TIB.

Highlight TIB.

Highlighting involves bringing the behavior to the client's attention by specifically observing and describing the behavior, related consequences affecting therapy or the therapy relationship, and providing a rationale (ideally linked to important goals of the client) to work on the behavior.

Assess the factors contributing to or maintaining TIB.

The clinician most commonly conducts a functional analysis (often referred to in DBT as a "chain analysis") of the chain of events associated with TIB, including (1) antecedents; (2) intervening emotions, physical sensations, thoughts, and actions; (3) the target TIB (frequency, duration, intensity); and (4) consequences, or events following TIB (internal, external, immediate and delayed).

Collaboratively solve problems contributing to or maintaining TIB.

The clinician roughly follows basic problem-solving steps (describe the problem, identify goals, brainstorm and evaluate potential solutions, implement solutions, and reevaluate; see Farmer & Chapman, 2016; Linehan, 2015; Nezu & Nezu, 2012) to collaboratively solve problems contributing to or maintaining TIB.

Seek a commitment to implement solutions.

The clinician uses motivational interviewing (see Miller & Rollnick, 2012) or DBT commitment strategies (see Linehan, 1993a) as appropriate to seek a commitment from the client to implement the agreed-upon plan.

Collaboratively troubleshoot problems that might interfere with the plan.

The clinician and client collaboratively identify and proactively solve problems or barriers that might interfere with the execution or effectiveness of the solutions/plans. Such factors may often include (1) lack of understanding of the skills/solutions; (2) lack of willingness to implement the solutions; (3) forgetting, or failure to discriminate the appropriate situations in which to use the solutions; or (4) various logistical issues (see "missing links analysis" in Linehan, 2015).

limitations, I do not elaborate on each of these steps in this chapter. In the next section, I focus primarily on the process of observing limits, which includes identifying, highlighting, and targeting TIB as needed, as these steps are perhaps most relevant to the problems commonly arising in DBT phone coaching.

Observing Limits around Phone Coaching

Phone coaching is among the areas of therapy in which the clinician's limits are perhaps most relevant. Phone coaching involves the clinician offering extra time to the client between therapy sessions, often during personal time that would otherwise be spent interacting with family or loved ones, fulfilling other work obligations, or engaging in recreational or leisure activities. This is a significant commitment. Even if clients rarely call, the knowledge that a client could call at some point may change the way clinicians approach or organize their personal time (e.g., that third glass of wine may not be advisable when a clinician has a client in crisis who will likely call that evening). At times, a client's repeated or prolonged calls, texts, or e-mails may threaten to burn out the clinician. For these reasons, it is important for clinicians to observe, monitor, and be crystal-clear regarding their personal limits around phone coaching.

In Chapter 2, I discussed the importance of considering possible limits around phone coaching, and in Chapter 3, I discussed ways to orient the client to these limits. Here, the focus is on *observing limits*. Clarifying and observing limits are related but different processes (Chapman & Rosenthal, 2016; Linehan, 1993a). As I discussed in Chapter 3, clarifying limits involves orienting the client to any specific limits around frequency, timing, duration, or the nature/focus of phone coaching contact. Clarifying limits essentially involves providing the client with "rules" the clinician would like both parties to agree on. Observing limits, in contrast, involves attending to whether the client's behavior is remaining within the clinician's limits, discussing deviations from these limits with the client, and collaboratively solving problems (often following many of the steps in Table 8.1).

Identifying TIB Related to Clinician Limits

To effectively observe limits, the clinician must mindfully observe and describe how client behaviors fit within the clinician's limits. Sometimes, this is relatively straightforward. If the clinician has conveyed a limit of three calls per week, and the client calls a fourth time, this should be considered potentially TIB and addressed during the next session. Similarly, if the clinician has conveyed the message that the focus of phone coaching is on skills, and the client refuses to discuss skills, this potentially TIB should fall outside the clinician's limits.

At other times, conflicts between client behavior and clinician limits is less clear. I once saw a client who never called too frequently and was pleasant, willing to talk about skills, and expressed gratitude for our calls. This client, however, spoke extremely slowly and frequently paused at length. His affect was despondent, and his responses to my suggestions were fairly noncommittal (e.g., "OK, I guess I'll try . . ."). As a result, I had difficulty getting off the phone, as I was worried that our calls were not as helpful as they could be. I also felt guilty about rushing our calls, given his level of distress combined with his gratefulness for my help. I did not notice at first, but our calls had been becoming longer and longer, to the point where we were regularly on the phone for about 30 minutes (well beyond my limits). I began to feel frustration and dread when I saw the client's number on my call display. At this point, I knew something was up. I used my frustration and dread as cues that TIB was occurring, suggesting that I needed to observe limits. With the help of my consultation team, I realized that the TIB in this case was primarily my own in two key ways. First, I was not managing the phone calls effectively. Some solutions to this problem involved (1) effective strategies to speed things up and conduct skills coaching in view of the client's depressive affect and behavior, (2) accepting the reality that we had not accomplished what I had hoped and ending the calls anyway, and (3) raising these issues with the client in session, so that we could collaboratively determine how to make our calls more effective. Second, I took a long time to notice this TIP pattern. To solve this problem, I paid closer attention to my emotional reactions when the client called (as well as during calls). I also kept closer track of the length of our calls, so I could catch a pattern of longer calls earlier in the process. As I hope this example illustrates, identifying TIB related to clinician limits requires mindfulness, both of external (e.g., length or frequency of calls, client behavior) and internal events (the clinician's emotions and thoughts). Exercise 8.1 includes a brief clinical example and exercise in identifying potential TIB and limit-pushing behavior.

EXERCISE 8.1 Identifying Potentially Therapy-Interfering or Limit-Pushing Behavior

Please read this vignette imagining you are in this situation: Imagine that you are seeing a client named Joan. Joan calls you at 11:30 P.M. and states in a loud and teary voice that her boyfriend broke up with her earlier that day. She says that she just knew this was going to happen and reminds you that she had really only agreed not to kill herself if her relationship with the boyfriend worked out. She says she is feeling intense despair, and that she has been lying in bed all day, having had about five drinks and a couple of Ativans in the early afternoon. Joan says she hasn't done anything to harm herself, but that she is feeling very suicidal. When you ask her what skills she has tried already to cope with this situation, she exclaims, "All you ever want to talk about is skills! No skill is going to fix this! The love of my life has just left me, and I'm totally devastated, and you want to talk about skills!? I thought I could count on you." You take some time to validate the client's concerns about skills and feelings about the breakup and listen empathetically as Joan speaks for the next 15 minutes about her feelings about the relationship ending. When you gently suggest that Joan try out some distress tolerance skills before going to bed, Joan says that she "doesn't think she's going to need those skills anymore." You query this statement, stating that you would like to work with her to reduce her suicide risk. Joan refuses to talk about this, stating that you are only concerned about your own liability, and hangs up the phone.

Practice Identifying Potential TIB Related to Clinician Limits and Devise a Plan

1. Imagine you are in this situation. Observe and describe your emotional reactions, thoughts, and any bodily sensations or urges arising in response to these interactions. Consider what information your internal reactions might be providing (i.e., the "wisdom" or value of your reactions).

2. Write down which of Joan's behaviors you believe go beyond your limits.

3. Write down how Joan's behaviors may are therapy interfering, in that they (a) make it difficult to conduct phone coaching, (b) hamper her progress in therapy, and/or (c) negatively affect the therapy relationship.

4. Devise a plan for what your next steps might be in view of possible issues of risk and how you might address TIB and observe limits (if applicable) in the next therapy session.

Highlighting TIB and Behaviors That Push the Clinician's Limits

Highlighting TIB simply means that the clinician should bring the TIB to the client's attention. The clinician raises the issue of TIB in a behaviorally specific manner, describing the behavior and its effect (or potential effect) on therapy or the therapy relationship, or its lack of fit with clinician limits. Ideally, the clinician highlights phone-coaching TIB in a clear, direct, and nonjudgmental manner. Highlighting allows the clinician and the client to get on the same page regarding a problem that they ideally will work on collaboratively and use as a therapeutic opportunity.

Highlighting phone-coaching TIB, however, is not always easy. Some clients are sensitive to feedback about their behavior generally and their phone-coaching behavior more particularly. This is understandable, as clients seeking phone coaching are reaching out for help, often when they are most distressed. I once worked with Julio, who initially was extremely reluctant to call me. After some practice calls, however, he became more comfortable with calling me. Over time, his rate of calling increased to the point where Julio was calling more than I could or wanted to manage. I realized that I needed to bring this issue up with him. I gently broached the topic, stating:

> "I'm really glad you've become comfortable with calling me, and I think we're doing some great work on the phone. We're figuring out how you can use skills from group to manage tough situations. I have noticed, however, that you've been calling me every day over the past few weeks. While I really want to help you, I can't keep up the daily contact. I don't even talk to my family every day if I can help it! I have a busy life, and it's hard to juggle my priorities and fit in all of these calls. I think we need to talk about how to make phone coaching work best for both of us. Would you be willing to talk about that?"

Julio was willing to talk about it, but he appeared increasingly frustrated, eventually exclaiming, "Fine, I just won't call you!" When I assessed this reaction, it became clear that he felt embarrassed and ashamed that he was intruding on my life. Indeed, at the beginning of therapy, he was reluctant to call out of concern that he would be bothering me or taking up too much of my time. Once we understood why this conversation was so difficult for him, we could move forward and find ways to make phone coaching work best for both of us.

A few guidelines can make the highlighting process smoother and more effective. First, highlighting is most effective when it is *behaviorally specific*. It is effective to describe client TIB in a specific, objective manner. This is much like using the mindfulness skill of "describe," mentioned above, as an antidote to judgment. In comparison with bringing up the behavior in a vague manner (e.g., "You're calling too often"), it can be more effective to be specific: "I've noticed that you're calling about five or six times per week." The clinician and client can work on specific behavior, such as the frequency of calling, the client's behavior during the call, and so on, but it is much harder to work on vague targets (e.g., "too much").

Second, highlighting should include a *rationale* for why it is important to address the TIB. The clinician might, for example, explain that he will not be able to sustain such frequent calls. When providing a rationale, I urge clinicians to focus on their own limits rather than on assumptions about the client's pathology. It may be easy to pathologize a client who calls, texts, or e-mails too often; gets upset with the clinician on the phone; is hard to get off the phone with; and the like. Clinicians might feel like suggesting that the client is too dependent or is resistant to change, noncooperative, or something else negative. Instead, when the client's calling negatively affects the clinician, it often is most effective to be direct about this problem. I have found that clients generally respond well to honest, genuine discussions of clinician limits. In addition, clients may be more willing to engage in such discussions and collaboratively solve the problem if the clinician links the problem behavior to the effectiveness of therapy. Ultimately, if the clinician is stressed, therapy is probably going to be less effective at helping the client reach his or her goals.

Employing Flexibility and Stretching Limits

Although clinician limits may seem clear from the beginning, limits can change. From a dialectical perspective, clinician limits can be both rigid and flexible, fixed and changeable. Several personal and professional factors can influence clinicians' limits around phone coaching, such as changes in the clinician's workload, professional and personal support available to the clinician, stress and life transitions (e.g., having babies and being sleep-deprived for a long time made me a lot less willing to take nighttime calls), and the history and quality of the therapy relationship. My willingness to be available for phone coaching generally increases when I am less overwhelmed with work, have a good balance of work and personal activities, and am not traveling too frequently. I am also more willing to engage in phone coaching when calls seem helpful and clients are willing to discuss and try skills. When there are persisting difficulties in the therapy relationship, the client does not appear willing to discuss or try skills, and I am receiving frequent calls, my willingness to be available decreases.

Years ago, I worked in a garment factory, in the seedy basement (i.e., sweat-shop) of a building in downtown Vancouver. My job was to make buttons. For nearly 8 hours a day (with two 15-minute coffee breaks and one 30-minute lunch break), I used a press machine to stamp fabric into the tops of little metal buttons. The expectation was that I would produce a certain number of buttons per shift. This was part of the job, and I agreed to it. Fortunately, it was a temporary job. Otherwise, instead of writing this book today, I would probably be languishing somewhere in long-term psychiatric care. Phone coaching is not like working in a factory, where the worker must produce a certain number of buttons. There is no reason clinicians need to be available for a certain number of calls of a certain duration per week. Phone coaching limits are more fluid than factory productivity expectations, and it is important for clients to know this fact. While clients often can expect their clinicians to be available weekly for standard 50-minute individual therapy sessions, clinician availability and willingness to engage in phone coaching can vary. When clinicians' limits change, it is crucial to orient clients to any changes as well as the associated rationale.

Just as some factors might make a clinician less willing to be available, other factors might suggest the need to *stretch limits* for a period (Linehan, 1993a). Stretching limits typically involves temporarily being more available to help and support the client. In terms of phone coaching, this might involve the clinician being available for more frequent or longer calls, getting back to the client more quickly, or providing greater flexibility around electronic communication. Clinicians might consider stretching their limits under a few key circumstances: (1) when the client is experiencing a stressful or difficult time and requires more support than usual; (2) when the client is experiencing prolonged crisis, and regular contact may reduce the risk of self-harm; or (3) when the client is making progress and the clinician wishes to reinforce this by temporarily providing extra contact (assuming such contact is a reinforcer). There are other considerations, but I would suggest that these are the three primary circumstances in which to consider stretching limits. When a clinician considers stretching limits around phone coaching, I recommend that she or he follow the steps discussed below.

Consider the Potential Pros and Cons of Stretching Limits

Do the potential benefits to the client or the therapy relationship outweigh the potential downsides or costs? Will limit stretching help to reduce serious or critical risk? Are there alternatives that might also help reduce risk? When risk is high, stretching limits should be simply one part of a broader plan to address and manage risk. Increased clinician availability should never be the *only* plan or solution to high-risk situations.

Clarify and Describe the New Limits and the Associated Rationale to the Client

Whenever limits are stretched, it is important to orient the client to the new limits and describe the clinician's rationale for stretching limits. Here is an example:

> "I know you've been going through an incredibly hard time since your girlfriend left you. You're barely holding on, feeling isolated and lonely, and thinking a lot about suicide. I think it makes sense for me to be a little more available during this time. I'm willing to take a couple of extra calls per week, and if you'd like, we could have an extra session this week and next week. I think a little extra support might help you get through this trying time and give us a chance to strategize about ways to help you rebuild some of what you have lost in the long run."

Orient the Client to the Time-Limited Nature of Limit Stretching

Limit stretching should almost always be temporary. There are a few key reasons for this. First, clinicians who stretch their limits for an indeterminate period run the risk of burnout, and having a clear timeline helps to reduce this risk. I am much more willing to stretch limits, throw myself into the process, and be as helpful as possible to my client if I know that things will go back to normal within, for example, a couple of weeks. Second, having a time limit can help the clinician avoid reinforcing crisis behavior with increased availability. When a time limit is in place, extra support and contact will cease regardless of whether the client continues to experience ongoing crises; thus, extra availability is not contingent on the continuation of the crisis. Third, as mentioned in a previous chapter, time limits facilitate effective, efficient work. When the clinician and client know that extra help and support will only occur for the next 2 weeks, both parties know that they need to get to work. In this case, the client ideally will be more motivated to make changes than if the period of limit stretching were indeterminate. Below is an example of how a clinician might discuss the time-limited nature of limit stretching:

> "I'm willing to have these extra calls and sessions for the next 3 weeks. I should let you know, though, that I won't be able to keep this up for longer than 3 weeks, given my workload and schedule. We're both going to have to work hard to help you find the skills you need to cope with what you're going through, and to do some extra problem solving to help build your life back up again. I know you're feeling terribly sad and devastated right now, and I imagine 3 weeks doesn't seem like much time, but it's the best I can do, and we're going have to make the most of our time."

Managing Contingencies Effectively

The effective management of contingencies is a crucial element of addressing challenges in phone coaching. Contingency management is a broad set of behavioral interventions involving the modification of contexts in which target behaviors occur. Typically, contingency-management strategies modify antecedents or consequences associated with particular behaviors (Farmer & Chapman, 2016; Linehan, 1993a). There are many ways to use contingency management. For a more extensive discussion of these approaches, please see Farmer and Chapman (2016), Goldfried and Davison (2012), and Kazdin (2012). Two key ways to manage contingencies in therapy settings include the modification of consequences occurring within the therapy relationship, and the creation of reinforcement, extinction, or punishment systems (Kohlenberg & Tsai, 1991; Linehan,

1993a). Working on the assumption that the reader has some familiarity with behavioral theory, I will discuss below a few key principles to keep in mind when managing contingencies regarding phone coaching.

Specify Behaviors to Increase or Decrease

Effective contingency management requires the delineation of behaviors to encourage or increase as well as behaviors to discourage or decrease. Common behaviors to increase include those that promote effective phone coaching and the use of skills in the client's everyday life. Examples could include the client calling the clinician at appropriate times for help with skills coaching; remaining within the clinician's limits regarding timing, duration, and frequency of calls (or electronic communication); expressing a willingness to discuss and use skills, among other possibilities. Behaviors to decrease include TIBs and actions that go beyond the clinician's personal limits, such as calls that are too frequent or too lengthy, excessive electronic communication, refusal to talk about or try skills, or other examples already discussed in this chapter.

When challenges arise in phone coaching, I suggest that clinicians put together a list of both desirable and undesirable behaviors. This not only clarifies behavioral targets but also might make the client's effective or skillful behaviors more salient. Indeed, I have often felt less frustrated after considering many of the effective or skillful things the client regularly does. I also find it helpful to remind myself of the key DBT assumption that "clients are doing the best they can" (Linehan, 1993a).

Use Reinforcement Selectively to Increase or Decrease Behaviors

Clinicians should ideally use contingency-management strategies to selectively decrease unwanted behaviors and increase desired behaviors. Perhaps the most straightforward way to do this is to make use of differential reinforcement procedures. *Differential reinforcement of other behavior (DRO)* involves providing reinforcement when a particular behavior does not occur. In the case of a client who is calling too frequently, the clinician might avoid reinforcing extra calls that go beyond therapeutic limits (e.g., by not answering, getting off the phone quickly, reminding the client that she or he is not available for another call), and provide reinforcement when she goes for a period without calling.

A related procedure, *differential reinforcement of alternative behavior (DRA)* involves providing reinforcement contingent on the client's engagement in some alternative, desired behavior. Consider a client who has been expressing frustration and refusing to talk about skills. The clinician might end calls earlier when the client is unwilling to talk about skills and provide more time and attention when the client collaboratively discusses skills. As another example, if a client has been overusing phone coaching for support and not accessing natural support networks, the clinician might consider ways to reinforce the client's seeking of alternative social support and spending time with friends or loved ones.

To effectively use DRO or DRA, the clinician should understand what factors increase or maintain behavior for his or her individual client. For some clients, extra contact or time with the therapist is an effective reinforcer, and for others the opposite is true. For some clients, the clinician highlighting progress or praising the client is an effective reinforcer, and for other clients praise has no effect on their behavior or even functions as punishment. For guidance on the range of clinician behaviors that could be used as reinforcers, consider consulting Kohlenberg and Tsai (1991) or Farmer and Chapman (2016) as well as some suggestions in Chapter 8. See also Pryor's *Don't Shoot the Dog* (2006).

Conceptualize Behavior in Terms of Process and Content

To effectively manage contingencies, the clinician must conceptualize therapy contact in terms of both *process* and *content*. Content has to do with what the client is saying or doing. The client, for example, might be saying that three phone calls per week is not enough for her or him, that therapy isn't working, that she or he is not willing to try the skills suggested, and so on. The content of hopeless thoughts would include the specific hopeless statements that the client is making about areas of her or his life, such as "I'll never get a job, have a relationship, or ever get married." It is, of course, important to pay attention to what the client is doing and saying, but it is difficult to manage contingencies unless the clinician also attends to process.

Process has to do with the *type of behaviors* in which the client is engaging. What type of behavior is happening when the client is saying that three phone calls is not enough for her or him? This could be considered the client expressing a need. Perhaps this is assertive behavior for the client. What about the client who says therapy isn't going to work?

This behavior could be considered "making hopeless statements." The client who states, "I don't want to try these skills" is basically expressing unwillingness to try a skill. The clinician focused on content might further assess these issues with the client: What makes her or him think therapy isn't going to work? Why is the client not willing to try a particular skill? Such assessment can be helpful, but a focus on prices helps the clinician attend to how these behaviors function for the client. Is it possible that stating that therapy isn't going to work is negatively reinforced by avoidance of difficult topics, or positively reinforced by extra concern and attention from the clinician? A functional view of the therapy process opens the door to an exploration of how the client's behavior functions in the context of therapy (or in other contexts).

Awareness of process can help the clinician remember to consider these client behaviors in terms of effectiveness. The question here is: Would it be helpful for the client to engage in more or less of this behavior? This question will help highlight which types of contingency-management strategies to use. If too much of a behavior (a behavioral excess) is occurring, then therapy strategies might focus on extinction or aversive procedures. In contrast, if an effective behavior is not occurring frequently enough, then strategies might focus on shaping, skills training, and positive or negative reinforcement.

Often, maintaining awareness at the level of process also can help clinicians to avoid becoming mired in the details of the content presented by the client, and reinforcing potentially problematic behaviors. A supervisee once described challenging interactions with her client. The client called for phone coaching but refused to try any skills and kept repeating that they were not getting to the most important issues in therapy. She stated that she wasn't making enough progress, that the clinician should stop talking about the fact that she's late every session, and that she has just gotten worse since she began therapy. Now, according to what has been presented in previous chapters, it should be clear that these are not phone coaching topics. Concerns about therapeutic progress are best addressed in individual therapy, where there is enough time to assess and address the issues. Brief heart-to-heart discussions of the therapy relationship can be helpful, but this client's calls tended to take a different turn.

Unfortunately, the clinician's worry about the client's concerns led her to become mired in the content of what the client was saying. She spent 45 minutes on the phone, trying to get the client to agree to try a skill and to convince her that therapy can be helpful and that she is willing to work on topics the client wants to address. Both the client and the clinician ended the call feeling frustrated. Apparently, this client had been improving, but she still often complained about therapy and said it wasn't working. When I assessed what the clinician typically did when the client complained about therapy (or about having to talk about being late), it became clear to me that the clinician talked a lot, inquired extensively about the client's concerns, and tried to encourage the client to continue. In fact, she increased her activity, talking, and expression of concern and caring specifically when the client complained. We hypothesized that the client may be receiving more positive (attention, time, support) and negative (avoidance of difficult emotions or topics) reinforcement when she complained than when she engaged in more collaborative, therapy-enhancing behavior.

Our solutions to this scenario involved several changes. First, the clinician reoriented the client to the structure of the phone calls and informed her that, if the client is willing to discuss skills, the clinician is willing to spend time on the phone (the other side of the coin being that calls would end if the client was unwilling to discuss skills). Second, the clinician halted "big" discussions about topics such as whether therapy is working and deferred these for individual therapy sessions. Third, the clinician looked for opportunities to reinforce active, skills-oriented engagement in phone coaching. When the client expressed willingness to talk about skills, was collaborative and cooperative, and so on, the clinician provided a little more time for the client to talk and increased her use of warmth and validation. Fourth, the clinician took the client's concerns about therapy seriously but (during in-person sessions) inquired whether the client might be avoiding difficult topics (such as the work they were doing on making new connections with coworkers).

Being Dialectical about TIB

Dialectical theory helps the therapist remember that therapy and phone coaching are transactional. The clinician behavior influences the client's behavior and vice versa. If the client is calling too often or engaging in unpleasant behaviors on the phone, it is quite likely that the clinician's behavior has something to do with this. I have found that taking this perspective helps me avoid blaming clients when they push my limits. I try to identify transactional aspects of the therapy system, including both my behavior and that of the client, that need to be changed to make phone coaching more effective for me and the client. As mentioned earlier in the chapter, dialectical theory also can help the clinician seek the wisdom in the client's apparently dysfunctional behavior. From a dialectical perspective, there is always truth or wisdom in both sides of opposing positions. When the TIB disrupts phone coaching or the therapist's limits are pushed, the challenge is for the clinician and client to seek the wisdom in each other's perspective. In addition, dialectical theory can help the therapist strike a balance between flexibility (e.g., extending limits) and rigidity (e.g., observing and maintaining limits) in phone coaching.

Summary

In summary, several key principles and strategies can help clinicians effectively manage or even prevent challenges arising during phone coaching. Some key principles include maintaining a mindful, nonjudgmental, and functional view of TIB. It is also helpful to view TIB systemically, dialectically, and as an opportunity to learn new things or address important areas that may cut across other domains of the client's life. Several key steps in managing TIB include (1) identifying TIB, (2) highlighting the behavior, (3) assessing factors contributing to TIB, (4) collaboratively problem solving, (5) seeking a commitment to problem solutions, and (6) troubleshooting. The primary focus in this chapter was on how some of these steps apply to the process of observing limits.

Observing limits involves mindfully attending to, observing, and describing client behavior in relation to clinician limits. Observing limits can facilitate effective phone coaching and help the clinician avoid burnout. To effectively observe limits, clinicians must identify and highlight TIB when relevant, discuss limits clearly and directly with the client, and consider when and how to be flexible about limits (i.e., stretch limits). Effective contingency management can help the clinician manage and prevent challenges to phone coaching. In addition, a dialectical perspective holds that therapy is a transactional process and encourages the clinician to seek the wisdom in the client's perspective and balance flexibility and rigidity.

CHAPTER 9

Skill Generalization and the Development of Self-Coaching Skills

his final chapter focuses on ways to help the client become her or his own coach. As mentioned in earlier chapters, generalization of behavior learned in therapy to everyday life is the paramount goal of phone coaching. Ideally, following therapy, clients will no longer need phone coaching, will maintain what they have learned, and will guide themselves in applying effective skills in their everyday lives. This does not mean that the ultimate goal of therapy is for clients to cope completely alone and independently of others. I have yet to meet someone who can do this. One of our key dialectical assumptions in DBT is that identity is relational, and that we are all in engaged in transactional relationships with others. Recognizing that we are all interdependent and connected to others and determining when and how to seek support is a useful and generalizable skill. This chapter addresses strategies to facilitate generalization both during and after therapy, with a primary focus on skills coaching. Although this chapter comes at the end of the book, it would be useful to read it before or during the early stages of phone coaching. Even early in treatment, clinicians can help their clients learn to coach themselves in the use of effective skills to improve their lives, both over the short and the long term.

Orientation

Beginning early in treatment, clinicians will find it helpful to orient the client to the goal of generalization. The clinician might, for example, describe how one important therapy goal is for the client to use the skills learned in therapy to maintain and improve his or her quality of life well beyond the end of therapy. Providing this message early, ideally during the orientation to therapy, can set the stage for future work focusing on the transfer of skills to everyday life during therapy and to life beyond the end of therapy.

During these discussions, it can be effective to begin to establish norms and expectations. I expect my clients to make therapy a part of their everyday lives. This often involves actively doing homework and trying what they are learning in therapy in many relevant situations. Ideally, the client also will try skills in increasingly challenging or complex situations. It can be useful to convey these expectations, along with the rationale for them, early in treatment. In the example dialogue below, the clinician makes the points that (1) homework practice is important, (2) practicing skills in many relevant situations (including increasingly challenging ones) can facilitate generalization, and (3) the client will benefit from learning how to guide and coach her- or himself.

THERAPIST: The kind of therapy we are doing, DBT, is all about learning new things. This means you will be learning new coping skills and strategies to improve your life. I have found that the best way to learn these things is to practice them as much as you can on a regular basis. That's why an important part of this therapy involves doing homework between sessions.

CLIENT: I know what you're saying, but I've always hated homework. I have a hard time remembering to do stuff like that, and I'm already really busy.

THERAPIST: You're not alone there! A lot of people hate homework and have a hard time getting it done, especially when their lives are busy. Never fear, I think we can get around that problem. If we do, I think you'll learn things that will help you meet other obligations. You've mentioned that you have a hard time getting to work meetings on time and completing reports and paper work, etc. So, the fact that our therapy involves homework is good news; we'll be able to work on something that really seems to get in your way.

CLIENT: OK, I see your point. I could use help being more organized and that kind of thing.

THERAPIST: Great! You're lucky to be working with me, then. I've had to learn, sometimes the hard way, to get more organized myself! So, I think I can help you with that. Let me tell you the other good news. Research has found that doing homework between sessions improves outcomes. So, the more you do your homework, the better therapy will probably work for you.

CLIENT: OK, you're starting to sell me on the homework idea even though I hate the word "homework." I'll do my best.

THERAPIST: Good to hear. A lot of people hate the word "homework." You could call it "skills practice" if you want. But I'm all for learning to tolerate difficult words like "homework." Difficult words are everywhere. People speak them all the time.

CLIENT: Yeah, yeah, I know.

THERAPIST: So, to summarize, this therapy involves learning new things, and homework is there to help you practice those new things. I'm also hoping that, once our work is done, you will continue to use what you have learned in therapy to cope with difficult times and keep your life going well. To do that, you'll have to try the skills you're learning in as many situations as possible. You'll also need to learn when and how to use the skills and how to remember to use them when you need to.

CLIENT: That makes sense.

THERAPIST: Good! As an example, one of the skills that can really help with anxiety is to change the way you breathe. It would be important to try the new kind of breathing in as many anxiety-provoking situations as possible, or even in other situations, like when you're coping with pain or when you feel angry with someone. That way, you will not only get better at the skill, but you will learn to use it in lots of situations, maybe even in new or unexpected situations.

CLIENT: That's good, you know that anxiety is one of my major problems. Other people have tried to teach me that breathing stuff, but I guess I've only used it when I've been panicking.

THERAPIST: Right, and if that's the case, you might have a hard time using it in other situations. This whole process is a lot like learning to drive. If you want to become an excellent driver and one day take a road trip across the country, you might start by learning to drive in a quiet, safe neighborhood with an instructor, parent, or friend in the car with you. Remember how I mentioned that part of our therapy involves phone coaching—calling me for help if you're not sure which skill to use or how to use it?

CLIENT: Yeah, I remember that.

THERAPIST: Well, phone coaching is kind of like having an instructor in the car with you. As time goes on, you will no longer need to have someone else in the car. As you become more comfortable, you'll need to practice driving in busier areas with more streetlights, traffic, and different rules and signs. This will help you prepare yourself to go wherever you might want to go one day. That cross-country road trip will be within your reach! Eventually, just like driving, our goal is for you to use the skills you're learning in therapy if and when you need them to take yourself wherever you might want to go. To do that, you'll have to learn how to be your own coach. Is that something you're willing to work on?

CLIENT: I can work on that, but I don't think I'm ready right now. I'm barely getting comfortable with this whole idea of calling you. But I'm really not coping well on my own, so I'm willing to give it a try. To be honest, I'm a little afraid that I'm going to start relying on you too much, though. That might put me a step backward or something.

THERAPIST: OK, I'm glad you brought that up. If that starts to happen, we can talk about it. It would be normal to rely on me a bit more in the beginning. In the future, we can work on helping you use the skills with less help from me. Does that sound good?

CLIENT: Yes.

THERAPIST: I'm glad to hear that. The bottom line is that you will get a lot more out of therapy if you throw yourself in with both feet, work hard, and try to make our work an important part of your life. Not only that, but if you make therapy part of your life, I'm confident that the benefits will last for a long time after our work is done.

In this example, the clinician addresses a few key topics related to generalization. She emphasized the importance of homework practice to build skills, the use of skills in a variety of situations, and the need to become increasingly independent with the skills, ultimately becoming one's own coach. In doing so, she clearly provided a rationale for the importance of generalization and used commitment strategies to ensure that the client is onboard. The clinician also framed potentially TIB (difficulty completing homework) as an opportunity to learn new things that might further enhance the client's quality of life. Finally, the clinician clearly conveyed the importance of making therapy part of the client's everyday life.

Assessing and Conceptualizing Barriers to Generalization

Throughout therapy, it is useful to keep the goal of generalization in mind and to assess whether the client is using his or her skills regularly in relevant situations. Clients sometimes demonstrate skills effectively in the therapeutic environment but not in their everyday lives. Andre, for example, effectively managed frustration and anger in group-therapy sessions when he became annoyed with other clients, and in individual therapy, where he effectively used breathing skills and reframing to dampen his anger. He continued, however, to regularly report blow-ups at home, with his partner and their children. Assuming Andre had acquired the skills he needed to manage anger (including both emotion regulation [ER] skills and effective communication strategies), there are at least a couple of reasons as to why he may not have demonstrated these skills at home: (1) insufficient response generalization, (2) lack of variation in skills-training contexts, or (3) the suppression of skillful behavior by contextual factors (Farmer & Chapman, 2016).

Response generalization involves displaying learned skills in other applicable situations. In Andre's case, he may not have adequately transferred the behaviors learned in the therapy context to his everyday life at home. This may be because he has not learned to identify the situations at home where managing anger and communicating effectively are likely to result in reinforcement (e.g., more pleasant interactions with his partner and children, getting his needs met without conflict). If this is the case, the clinician might help Andre learn to discriminate situations in which these skills would be effective. He may, for example, need training to identify cues or situations associated with anger at home (suggesting that skills may be needed), physiological cues indicating that anger has increased, or cues suggesting that certain interpersonal skills may be effective (e.g., situations in which it may be effective to apologize for not completing a household task, or when simply listening to his partner without becoming defensive may be most effective).

Andre might also need more training or instruction in effective anger management and communication in heated situations, such as those occurring at home. This could involve bringing relevant triggers into the therapy room via imaginal rehearsal of situations occurring at home, role-play practice with the clinician playing the role of Andre's family members, or some combination of these or other approaches. The goal would be to make the situations in which Andre practices skills as similar as possible to his home environment, and to gradually have him practice at home under increasingly challenging situations.

Another reason for Andre's lack of skill use at home could be that contextual features in the home environment *suppress skillful behavior* (Farmer & Chapman, 2016). The presence of particular emotional states (very intense anger) or cognitions/rules (e.g., "Apologizing means I'm weak") could road-block effective anger management and communication strategies. In these cases, therapy might focus initially on strategies to dampen the intensity of Andre's anger or to develop and rehearse more effective thinking.

Andre's learning history in similar circumstances may also suppress skillful behavior. Andre may have, for example, experienced punishing consequences (e.g., his partner criticizing or chastising him) when he has tried to use breathing strategies or to take a brief time-out from conflict (usually helpful strategies). In this case, the clinician might focus on ways for Andre to respond to criticism and continue to cope effectively with anger.

Strategies to Facilitate Skills Generalization

Several key strategies can facilitate the generalization of skills to the client's natural environment and to life beyond the end of therapy. In the sections below, I discuss a few different approaches to generalization, including varied skills practice and stimulus control procedures. There are, of course, other approaches to generalization, but I have included those that are most consistent with and most commonly used in DBT. For the purposes of this section (and this chapter more generally), I will assume that clients already have acquired and strengthened relevant skills. Therefore, the focus is on transferring these skills to the natural environments rather than approaches to further build or strengthen skills.

Varied Skills Practice

Varied skills practice involves the practice of skills in as many relevant situations as possible. As suggested above, Andre may have needed to practice anger management and communication skills in situations more similar to what he encounters at home. Encouraging the client to practice skills in a broad range of situations can increase the chances that the target skillful behavior will occur automatically when needed, and help increase the range of contexts and stimuli that may occasion effective skill use. If a client has learned the DBT ER skill of problem solving, for example, the clinician might suggest the use of this skill to solve problems at work, at home, on transit, when setting financial goals, and so on. ER strategies such as paced breathing and opposite action can be effective for a variety of emotional states. The clinician, therefore, might encourage Andre to use these skills for varying intensities of anger as well as other emotions, such as sadness, guilt, and shame. Interpersonal effectiveness, distress tolerance, and mindfulness skills similarly can be applicable and practiced in many contexts.

Stimulus Control

Stimulus control strategies generally involve removing or modifying stimuli, introducing stimulus cues, and discrimination training, among other strategies (Farmer & Chapman, 2016). Incorporating stimulus control strategies into therapy and into life beyond the end of therapy can facilitate generalization. In behavioral terms, a behavior is under stimulus control when it occurs reliably in the presence of a particular stimulus but not in the absence of this stimulus. When clients like Andre have learned skills but do not display them in applicable situations, the skills might not have come under appropriate stimulus control. Stimulus control strategies often involve training the client to engage in skillful behavior in the context of stimuli encountered in relevant everyday situations. Such strategies can help strengthen skills, as clients making use of stimulus control may engage in more skills practice. Stimulus control also can help generalize skills to situations outside of the therapy context and to the period following the end of therapy.

Cue Elimination

Removing stimuli or antecedents for behavior, often referred to as *cue elimination,* involves removing the cues that occasion particular target behaviors (Farmer & Chapman, 2016). At times, the presence of particular cues in the client's environment may elicit problem behaviors and reduce the client's opportunity to use and practice behavioral skills. The client attempting to learn skills to reduce drug use, for example, would have difficulty doing so if she continued to spend a lot of time with drug-using friends or around drug paraphernalia. Removing or altering these stimuli can increase the chances that the client will engage in the types of skills learned in therapy as well as the ease of doing so. In DBT for substance-using patients, a common strategy within this category involves "burning bridges," or cutting off ties to drug-using friends and acquaintances, and avoiding situations in which drugs are to be found.

Cue Introduction or Modification

Stimulus control strategies also involve the *introduction of cues* for skillful behavior. Such cues can serve as reminders or prompts for the client to regularly practice relevant skills or use such skills in situations in which they are urgently needed. To facilitating ongoing practice, a client learning interpersonal effectiveness skills might prompt him- or herself to regularly practice the skills by scheduling reminders in his or her smartphone; writing notes or reminders about the skills on specific days of a calendar; placing notes, homework sheets, or other materials in strategic locations around the home; and so on. It is possible, of course, that the client may see a reminder but decide not to practice the skill. Failure to practice may be due to busyness, low motivation, willfulness, or other factors. Fortunately, DBT also includes skills to solve practical problems and barriers, enhance motivation, and increase willingness (Linehan, 2015). Therefore, it can be useful for the clinician and the client to troubleshoot the possibility that the client might disregard reminders, assess barriers such as motivation and willfulness, and devise plans to circumvent those barriers.

The following are some examples of ways in which cues may be introduced to elicit skill-related behavior:

- Joni had learned that at times the most effective way to manage interpersonal conflict was to gracefully take a time-out and practice distress tolerance skills before returning to the discussion. When she started to feel increasingly tense and angry, the first sign typically was tension in her jaw. She used that sensation as a cue to stop talking (she associated tension in the jaw with the need to temporarily "keep her mouth shut"), take a breath, and respectfully request a time-out from the discussion. Typically, this would occur at home, so she had some coping cards in her study reminding her of skills to use during these time-outs.

• Sam had overcome self-injury 6 months ago but still periodically struggled with strong urges to cut, particularly in the evenings when he was alone for prolonged periods or after he had a couple of drinks. As he typically had cut with either a kitchen knife or an old straight razor in his bathroom, he stuck red Post-it notes to the side of his kitchen knife block as well as to his bathroom mirror. Because he did not want visitors to know the purpose of these Post-it notes, they were blank. He had trained himself to associate red Post-it notes with the need to use distress tolerance skills in order to avoid "red-lining."

• Elizabeth had made a lot of progress in treatment for her panic disorder and agoraphobic behaviors. She now regularly gets out of the house, seeing friends, going to coffee shops, and so on. At times, she still feels fearful prior to these activities and has urges to simply stay in her house. She also sometimes fears the possibility of a panic attack when she experiences certain body sensations, such as increased heart rate and body temperature. During exposure therapy, she learned (1) to accept and tolerate her feelings of anxiety, (2) that physical symptoms do not always predict an impending panic attack, and (3) that public places and gatherings were not particularly dangerous (even if she were to have a panic attack). She came to associate the word "accept" with acceptance of her sensations of anxiety and the words "So what?" (as in "So what if I have a panic attack?") and "safety" with the idea that feared situations are probably safe. She programmed these words to pop up on her smartphone as reminders each day.

To further facilitate generalization, it can be useful to orient the client thoroughly to the rationale for these stimulus control strategies and provide instruction regarding how to continue to use stimuli to occasion skillful behavior (Farmer & Chapman, 2016). Ideally, for example, the client may develop a regimen of stimulus control that she or he can sustain beyond the end of therapy.

Therapy Reminders

Another way to introduce helpful cues into the client's everyday life is to make use of *therapy reminders*. Therapy reminders can include reminders about therapy, about the clinician, and about what the client has learned. It is quite possible, and likely disturbingly common, that clients will proceed through therapy, learn many new and helpful things, and then later have a hard time recalling what they actually did in therapy. I have worked with several clients who have had previous, long-term therapy and still have difficulty remembering the clinician's name, the type of treatment they received, or what was most helpful about therapy. At times, such clients may report vague recollections that they learned a few coping skills or found the relationship with the clinician to be helpful in their path to recovery. For clients to become their own therapeutic coaches, I believe it is important for them to develop more specific, elaborate, and useful memories of their experiences in therapy.

Perhaps the most common example of a therapy reminder in DBT is the provision of an audio-recording of therapy sessions to clients. Although this is certainly not a requirement for DBT adherence, many DBT clinicians regularly provide such recordings. In the past, this may have involved the use of a tape recorder, but it is more common now for the clinician (or client) to record sessions digitally and provide an electronic copy in some way. When these recordings are provided, it is important to orient the client to potential risks to confidentiality or issues that may arise while listening to therapy recordings. In terms of confidentiality, I recommend that clinicians caution clients to save therapy recordings in a secure, encrypted, password-protected manner and to avoid sharing them with others or uploading them in any way to social media. Although I have nearly always found that providing audio-recordings facilitates therapy, at times, clients may listen to a recording and become distressed, start to second-guess or have negative interpretations about themselves or the clinician's behavior, and so on. It is helpful to let clients know that, should this happen, they are welcome to raise any emerging issues or concerns in the next therapy session. The major advantages of providing an audio-recording are as follows:

- Clients often forget important things that they have learned in specific sessions. Hearing exactly what was said and done can help consolidate clients' memories of therapy and firm up any lessons they might have learned.

- When therapy has included a significant focus on exposure-oriented interventions, listening to session recordings may provide additional exposure and enhance the effective treatment. Indeed, in prolonged exposure therapy for trauma, clients typically listen daily to exposure trials conducted during therapy sessions (Foa & Rothbaum, 2001).

- Clients also may learn how to coach themselves in skills by listening to how the clinician does this in session. Individual DBT sessions often involve a variety of therapy strategies, including coaching, feedback, and suggestions regarding skill use. Ultimately, the hope is that clients will learn to be their own coaches. Assuming that the clinician is at least somewhat skillful at coaching, he or she may serve as a model for the client's own self-coaching skills.

Another specific example of a therapy reminder is the use of *extinction reminders* (Bouton & Brooks, 1993) in the treatment of anxiety disorders. Theory and research suggest that, even following successful exposure treatment for a phobia or other type of fear, the renewal of such fears is common (Bouton, 2000, 2004; Craske et al., 2014). This is often because when we learn to be afraid of something, this learning often generalizes to a variety of contexts in which we might encounter the feared object or situation. In contrast, learning that the object or situation is safe tends to be fairly context-dependent. A client might learn that it is safe to play with a spider in the therapy office but still panic at the sight of one crawling up her or his wall at home.

Particularly relevant to the issue of generalization beyond therapy, as time passes and life circumstances change, the safety learning that occurred in the therapy context may not adequately generalize to new life contexts. As a result, fears and anxiety may return. To reduce the likelihood of this problem, extinction reminders are cues that remind the client of the learning that took place during exposure therapy. An extinction reminder might simply be a visual or auditory cue that the client can use in applicable situations, for example, while interacting with other people (for a socially anxious client), spending time in nature (for a client afraid of insects), and so on. Extinction reminders also could include coping self statements, words (e.g., "calm," "peace," "release," or "relax") that have become paired with relaxation or safety, among other stimuli. As exposure-oriented procedures often are used for a variety of clinical problem areas, it is helpful to consider extinction reminders for clients suffering from problems other than anxiety disorders or fears. For a discussion of the use of extinction reminders in the treatment of substance use problems, for example, see Rosenthal and Kutlu (2014).

Therapy reminders also can include reminders yoked to particular skills, or more general reminders of therapy, the clinician, and key skills the client has learned. One helpful way to both introduce therapy reminders and to say good-bye effectively to clients at the end of therapy is to write a letter describing and summarizing the type of work that was done in therapy, the skills the client seemed to find most effective, and any behavioral plans to manage difficult or high-risk situations. The letter also might comment on the types of skills the client used in challenging situations involving phone coaching.

As another example, when I lead DBT skills training groups, I send clients weekly homework reminders, summarizing the skills we covered that week, the mindfulness practice we engaged in, and the specific homework assigned for that week. Each reminder also includes a quote that is generally relevant to DBT or specifically applicable to the skills that I taught that week. I e-mail these homework reminders to current group members as well as to previous group members who have asked to remain on my e-mail list. Over the past 10 years or so since I began sending these reminders, only a few previous clients have asked to be removed from the list. Many clients have expressed gratitude, stating that the ongoing e-mails have encouraged them to continue to practice their skills. I also send birthday wishes to previous clients, even years after therapy has ended, and I have found that they almost uniformly appreciate this, and I suspect that these birthday wishes serve at least as brief reminders of therapy.

It also can be useful to take steps to enrich and expand the client's memories of therapy. Quotes, stories, or even inside jokes shared between the clinician and the client can help to enrich good-bye letters from the clinician. Some clients may also benefit from having a photograph of the therapy room or of the clinician. If the client often drank a particular type of tea in the clinician's office or was exposed to particular odors from potpourri or flowers and so on, it could be helpful for the client to remember these and use them to recall the experience of therapy later on. Elaborative rehearsal of therapy memories including many stimulus elements may facilitate recall. Researchers have suggested that this is because memories are stored and activated through a process of spreading activation, involving many different neural networks and nodes, capturing sensory, motor, and other experiences associated with the memory (Anderson, 1983).

Developing Self-Coaching Skills

In this section, I emphasize strategies clinicians can use during phone coaching to help clients develop self-coaching skills. Much like any other set of skills, self-coaching includes a group of behaviors that can be learned, strengthened, and generalized to a variety of applicable situations. Just as a client learning assertiveness skills might start small by learning to make eye contact and progress toward using effective strategies to assert her or his needs, self-coaching skills can be shaped, reinforced, and expanded.

Often, learning these or other skills begins with the process of *shaping*. Shaping involves reinforcing successive approximations of a desired behavior or set of behaviors (Ferguson & Christiansen, 2008). To effectively use shaping principles, it is helpful for the clinician to identify and operationalize the ultimate target behavior or behaviors. In the case of self-coaching, the ultimate desired behaviors often vary from client to client but also have some common elements. Below is an example of five reasonable behavioral targets for the majority of clients.

1. The client specifically *observes and describes* the current situation contributing to emotional distress, as well as thoughts, physiological sensations, emotional states, and related urges. The client self-validates, emphasizing how and why her or his experiences might be understandable given the current situation, past learning, or personal characteristics.

2. The client *identifies the general category* of skills (e.g., ER, interpersonal effectiveness, mindfulness, or distress tolerance) as well as the *specific skills* that may be most useful. Often, some combination of the skills is most useful; thus, ideally, the client has learned to identify when this is the case.

3. The client *knows why, when, and how to use the skill* or seeks appropriate guidance, either by reviewing material from therapy, or

perhaps by seeking support or suggestions from someone in her or his natural social network.

4. The client uses strategies, as needed, to *encourage or motivate* her- or himself to use skills. This may involve strategies such as considering the pros and cons of using skills (one of the distress tolerance skills; Linehan, 2015) and coping self statements, among other approaches, in addition to seeking encouragement from others.

5. When skills do not seem to be working as hoped, the client *troubleshoots effectively*. This may involve brainstorming alternative skills, reevaluating or reconceptualizing the problem situation, seeking help or support from others, and the like.

This may seem like a tall order for some clients. Many of these targets, however, already are addressed in the standard course of skills training in DBT. The client primarily has to learn how to bring these behaviors together in challenging situations. Much of the work done during phone coaching involves helping the client do just that. The challenge, then, is for the clinician to help the client to engage in these behaviors with decreasing therapeutic support.

Directly Teaching the Client Self-Coaching as a Skill

Although "self-coaching skills" are something I just made up for this book and are not part of standard DBT skills training, it can be effective to teach coaching as we do other skills in DBT. In addition, the DBT skills training manual (Linehan, 2015) does include self-management skills, which can be very helpful in this regard. In addition, in Chapter 5, I discussed a variety of skills training and coaching principles and strategies, which can be applied to the teaching of self-coaching. Essentially, the clinician should first identify and describe the skills the client is learning along with an associated rationale for learning them. An example is presented in the dialogue below:

THERAPIST: As we've discussed, we've used phone coaching, skills coaching during our therapy sessions, and homework review in skills training group to help you use skills you're learning in therapy in your everyday life. You've learned a lot of DBT skills, but coaching yourself is another important skill to learn. Self-coaching involves coaching yourself in skills you need in the moment. We all need to be able to coach ourselves in skills, especially when life is really hard. Does that sound reasonable?

CLIENT: Yeah, but it makes me anxious to have to do that without you.

THERAPIST: I know, and we're not there yet, but if we get started soon, I think you'll feel a lot more confident once therapy's over.

CLIENT: OK.

THERAPIST: So, coaching yourself includes a few different things. First, you need to use mindfulness skills to observe and describe whatever situation you're in and notice that you need to use skills to help yourself. It can also be helpful to validate how you feel. Make sense?

CLIENT: Sounds like a good place to start.

THERAPIST: Good, next, you have to be able to figure out what type of skills could help. So, for example, if you're in a situation where you feel urges to hurt yourself or do something else that might make things worse, what skills would you consider?

CLIENT: Crisis survival strategies?

THERAPIST: Right on! Next, you'd need to know when, how, and why to use the skill. So, for the crisis survival strategies, give me an example of how you could use distraction to ride out a painful situation.

CLIENT: I think my best go-tos for that are TV or just getting the heck out. Going somewhere like the coffee shop down the street or walking in the park or something. Getting away from where I'm miserable seems to get my mind off things for a little while.

THERAPIST: Exactly, that has helped you many times in the past. Another part of coaching yourself is motivating or encouraging yourself when you really don't feel like using skills, think they won't work, or get really demoralized.

CLIENT: That still happens, but I wish it didn't.

THERAPIST: I know, and it might continue to happen from time to time. Remember what we came up with that you could say to yourself when you get really demoralized?

CLIENT: This too shall pass, or I'm already like 100 steps up the staircase, or something like that.

THERAPIST: I remember those. What else? What about if you don't feel like using skills?

CLIENT: Even though it's annoying, it always helps when you say, "That's a thought, not necessarily a fact. Let's just try it out and see what happens." I can get stuck thinking things won't work, and then I don't do anything.

THERAPIST: Perfect, how about you write that down? OK, so the last step is to be able to troubleshoot—figure out what to do if skills don't work or if something gets in your way. Alright, to summarize, coaching yourself involves at least five basic steps, and we're going to work on these over the next few months.

Reinforcing and Shaping Self-Coaching Skills

The clinician should seek opportunities to reinforce instances of self-coaching. As mentioned in Chapter 3, effective therapeutic coaches are keen observers of client behavior. Whenever the client engages in behaviors that will ultimately support self-coaching, the clinician must notice these behaviors and ideally provide positive feedback or reinforcement. Although a discussion of the use of reinforcement in therapy is beyond the scope of this chapter or book (for a more detailed discussion of contingency management and therapeutic reinforcement, see Farmer & Chapman, 2016; Kohlenberg & Tsai, 1991; Linehan, 1993a), the clinician may use reinforcement in several ways. Below are a few examples:

- Praise
- Increased responsivity, warmth, or enthusiasm
- Increased use of validation
- Increased time permitted for the client to talk about preferred topics
- Reduced time for the client to talk about nonpreferred topics
- Comments on the client's positive progress
- Comments linking the client's behavior to valued goals
- Increased (or decreased, for clients whose behavior is negatively reinforced by the reduction of session time) session time
- Tangible reinforcers, such as stickers, prizes, and so on.

As the goal is to facilitate the generalization of skills and the development of self-coaching abilities, the clinician may opt for the more natural forms of reinforcement, as these are more logically connected with the client's behavior and likely to facilitate generalization of effective behavior beyond therapy (Kohlenberg & Tsai, 1991). In addition, using shaping principles, the clinician would expect the client to demonstrate more self-coaching behaviors over time before providing the same degree of reinforcement.

Dragging Out New Behavior

Another way to help clients develop self-coaching skills is to *drag out new behavior*. Dragging out new behavior involves prompting the client to engage in new, skillful behavior (Linehan, 1993a). This most commonly involves prompting and encouraging the client to practice a skill in the moment, or throwing the ball in the client's court and asking her or him to come up with solutions to a problem. DBT is a learning-oriented therapy, and it is difficult to learn new skills without actively practicing them. Coaching and guidance on the client's active use of self-coaching behaviors, both in individual therapy sessions (and group skills training) and during phone coaching, can help strengthen and refine these behaviors and encourage their generalization to everyday life. This is why dragging out new behavior is required for adherence in all DBT individual therapy and DBT skills training sessions.

During phone coaching, it is helpful for the clinician to look for opportunities to drag out new, self-coaching-related behaviors, keeping in mind the five targets discussed above. Following shaping principles, the clinician might use this approach more often as therapy progresses. Below is an example of a portion of a phone coaching session in which the clinician drags out a few of the five behaviors described above as important targets for clients learning to coach themselves.

THERAPIST: OK, so maybe start by describing what just happened, your sensations, emotions, thoughts, and urges.

CLIENT: Oh boy, this is so hard. I had left my e-mail open on my computer, and Ken saw a message from that guy I see at Starbucks every week. We talked about him, right?

THERAPIST: Yes, Mark, right?

CLIENT: Yeah, well I was out for a walk, and Ken read several of the messages. When I got home, he was all distant and quiet, and then he kind of exploded and came out and asked me if I was having an affair with Mark. I tried to explain that he was just a nice guy that I bumped into at Starbucks regularly, and we had sort of struck up a friendship and shared our e-mail addresses, but he started yelling at me. I have to say I was really effective. I didn't yell back, and I tried to listen as best I could. But he started crying, and I just couldn't handle it. I had to get out of there. At first, I was shocked and really anxious, but now I just feel sad and guilty.

THERAPIST: Gosh, that really sounds hard. Now, I want to have you practice a little self-validation here. How does it make sense that you feel sad and guilty?

CLIENT: I guess I'm sad because this whole thing really has hurt Ken. I'm also sad because this might change our relationship. I feel like I'm losing something.

THERAPIST: How about guilty?

CLIENT: Well, I feel guilty for hurting Ken. I know it looks fishy with Mark, and I would probably feel the same way if Ken was doing the same thing. I mean, I sort of have feelings for Mark, but it's nothing I would ever act on. It's just kind of nice to have a little spark and someone to look forward to chatting with every week at Starbucks.

THERAPIST: That makes perfect sense to me. So, dealing with this sadness and guilt, what skills come to mind?

CLIENT: Now that I've taken a breather, the emotions are not as strong, and I think I can tolerate them. I already sort of did some distress tolerance. I think maybe emotion regulation would be the best thing now before I go back to talk to Ken. Actually, maybe also some interpersonal effectiveness.

THERAPIST: Right on, that's exactly what I would've suggested! You really are catching on to how the skills can work. I'm impressed that you're able to do this so soon after the event and with all the strong emotions you're feeling. Which emotion regulation skills do you think might help most?

CLIENT: Oh God, there are just so many of them! I was already kind of mindful of my emotions, so I don't think I need any more of that right now. I guess opposite action?

THERAPIST: Let's think about that for a moment. When is opposite action usually most useful?

CLIENT: When the emotion is not justified? Like when it doesn't fit the facts?

THERAPIST: Exactly. So, do you think sadness and guilt fit the facts?

CLIENT: Guilt, definitely. I know I didn't do anything intentionally to hurt him, but the thing with Mark is almost like a bit of an emotional affair, and that doesn't fit my values. Not that I necessarily want to stop. . . .

THERAPIST: Yes, that does complicate things. But I think you are on the right track. So, when guilt is justified, what can you do?

CLIENT: It's not opposite action, so it must be something like accept it. Is that right?

THERAPIST: Yes, you could always use the skill of acceptance. You could also try to solve the problem. For guilt, solving the problem often involves apologizing, making amends, fixing whatever damage was caused, that kind of thing. How you do that is completely up to you and has to fit your values and your relationship with Ken. So, let's agree that you will give that some thought when you get off the phone with me.

CLIENT: OK, I can do that.

THERAPIST: What about sadness? Is sadness justified?

CLIENT: That's a hard one.

THERAPIST: How would you know?

CLIENT: Isn't it if I have lost something important or something?

THERAPIST: That's one type of situation that can justify sadness. But sometimes we might feel sad if someone else is hurt or in distress.

CLIENT: I do feel kind of sad for Ken, but to be honest, the sadness has more to do with the idea that our relationship is damaged and can't be fixed. So, I guess, I feel sad and kind of sick to my stomach because I think I'm losing something.

THERAPIST: I could imagine feeling the same way. It's not clear, however, that you actually have lost something yet, or that anything has been irreparably damaged. So, I might say that sadness about Ken being distressed fits the facts, but sadness about damage to the future of the relationship might not fit the facts right now. . . .

In this example, the clinician throws the ball into the client's court and drags out new behavior several times. In fact, the clinician rarely makes a suggestion without first encouraging the client to come up with one herself. This client was far along in therapy, having completed a full cycle of DBT skills training, so it would be reasonable to expect her to know most of the skills and to determine when to use them. This example, therefore, is most relevant for clients who are fairly far along in therapy.

The clinician prompted or dragged out at least four of the five target behaviors listed above. The clinician began by prompting the client to observe and describe the situation and related experiences and then encouraged the client to engage in some self-validation (target #1). Other behaviors that were prompted included the client identifying a general category of skills that could be helpful and zeroing in on a particular skill within that category (targets #2 and #3). The clinician provided some coaching regarding the opposite action framework and helped the client figure out whether emotions were justified and what to do about them (target #4). Notice, however, that the clinician did not help the client figure out what to say to Ken, how to repair the situation, and so on. Instead, the clinician prompted the client to do that work primarily on her own.

Being Dialectical about Generalization and Self-Coaching

Despite the focus in this chapter on increasing client independence with skills and skills coaching, dialectical theory helps the clinician remember that there is a balance between dependence and independence. Dialectical theory holds that identity is relational. It would be very hard to define our own identity without reference to the context in which we live, including people, places, things, and the broader world around us. The idea is that we are all part of a transactional system, and we are all connected in some way to the universe. From this perspective, independence is a myth. It is impossible to be completely independent or separate from others. We are all both separate and connected at the same time. In his book, *Being Peace*, Thich Nhat Hanh (1996) has described how a simple piece of paper contains all of the workers involved in making the paper, the food these workers have eaten, the sun and clouds (through rain) that have helped this food grow, the workers' ancestors, and so on. The idea that clients must manage their lives completely independently is misguided. At the same time, it is effective to help clients learn how to coach themselves and bring what they have learned into their everyday lives so that they can continue to benefit long after therapy has come to a close. From a dialectical perspective, some of this work could involve helping clients strike an effective balance of independence and dependence, such as by helping them learn how to help themselves and when and how to seek help from others.

Summary

In summary, phone coaching is one of many approaches to facilitate the generalization of skills and lasting treatment gains. This chapter covered several key strategies and concepts related to generalization, including the importance of orienting the client to the principle of generalization, assessing potential barriers to generalization, and a variety of strategies to facilitate generalization. Some strategies include encouraging the client to practice skills in a variety of contexts, the use of stimulus control procedures, and the creative use of therapy reminders. It is also important to help the client develop the ability to coach and guide her- or himself in effective skills. Self-coaching requires a variety of behaviors, such as observing and describing external and internal experiences; identifying effective skills; determining when, why, and how to use the skills; self-encouragement and motivation; and troubleshooting. Clinicians can facilitate the development of self-coaching skills by teaching these skills directly, using shaping and contingency management principles, and dragging out new behavior to allow the client to gain practice in coaching her- or himself. Throughout treatment, the hope is that the clinician also has served as an effective model for how to use skills coaching. A dialectical worldview helps the clinician remember that we are all both connected and separate, that complete independence is a misguided ideal, and that a life worth living involves helping ourselves and knowing when and how to seek help from others.

References

Abramowitz, J. S. (2013). The practice of exposure therapy: Relevance of cognitive-behavioral theory and extinction theory. *Behavior Therapy, 44,* 548–558.

Abramowitz, J. S., Deacon, B. J., & Whiteside, S. P. (2011). *Exposure therapy for anxiety: Principles and practice.* New York: Guilford Press.

American Psychological Association. (1997). APA statement on services by telephone, teleconferencing, and Internet. Retrieved from *www.apa.org/ethics/education/telephone-statement.aspx.*

Anderson, J. R. (1983). A spreading activation theory of memory. *Journal of Verbal Learning and Verbal Behavior, 22,* 261–295.

Andrews-Hanna, J. R. (2011). The brain's default network and its adaptive role in internal mentation. *The Neuroscientist, 18,* 251–270.

Barlow, D. H. (2011). *Unified protocol for transdiagnostic treatment of emotional disorders: Therapist guide.* New York: Oxford University Press.

Baumeister, R. F. (1990). Suicide as escape from self. *Psychological Review, 97,* 90–113.

Beck, A. T. (1979). *Cognitive therapy of depression.* New York: Guilford Press.

Beedie, C. J., & Lane, A. M. (2011). The role of glucose in self-control: Another look at the evidence and an alternative conceptualization. *Personality and Social Psychology Review, 16,* 143–153.

Ben-Porath, D. D. (2015). Orienting clients to telephone coaching in dialectical behavior therapy. *Cognitive and Behavioral Practice, 22,* 407–414.

Blakey, S. M., & Abramowitz, J. S. (2016). The effects of safety behaviors during exposure therapy for anxiety: Critical analysis from an inhibitory learning perspective. *Clinical Psychology Review, 49,* 1–15.

Bongar, B., Sheykhani, E., Kugel, U., & Giannini, D. (2015). The formal assessment of suicide risk. In U. Kamar (Ed.), *Suicidal behavior: Underlying dynamics* (pp. 202–212). New York: Routledge.

Bongar, B., & Sullivan, G. R. (2013). *The suicidal patient: Clinical and legal standards of care* (3rd ed.). Washington, DC: American Psychological Association.

Bouton, M. E. (2000). A learning theory perspective on lapse, relapse, and the maintenance of behavior change. *Health Psychology, 19*(1, Suppl.), 57–63.

Bouton, M. E. (2004). Context and behavioral processes in extinction. *Learning and Memory, 11,* 485–494.

Bouton, M. E., & Brooks, D. C. (1993). Time and context effects on performance in a Pavlovian discrimination reversal. *Journal of Experimental Psychology, Animal Behavior Processes, 19,* 165–179.

Canadian Psychological Association. (2006). Draft ethical guidelines for psychologists providing psychological services via electronic media. Retrieved from *www.cpa.ca/aboutcpa/committees/ethics/psychserviceselectronically.*

Chapman, A. L., & Gratz, K. L. (2016). *The DBT skills workbook for anger.* Oakland, CA: New Harbinger.

Chapman, A. L., & Rosenthal, M. Z. (2016). *Managing therapy interfering behaviors: Strategies from dialectical behavior therapy.* Washington, DC: American Psychological Association.

Choi-Kain, L. W., Zanarini, M. C., Frankenburg, F. R., Fitzmaurice, G. M., & Reich, D. B. (2010). A longitudinal study of the 10-year course of interpersonal features in borderline personality disorder. *Journal of Personality Disorders, 24*(3), 365–376.

Craske, M. G., Treanor, M., Conway, C. C., Zbozinek, T., & Vervliet, B. (2014). Maximizing exposure therapy: An inhibitory learning approach. *Behavior Research and Therapy, 58,* 10–23.

Crowell, S. E., Beauchaine, T. P., & Linehan, M. M. (2009). A biosocial developmental model of borderline personality: Elaborating and extending Linehan's theory. *Psychological Bulletin, 135*(3), 495–510.

Drude, K., & Lichstein, M. (2005). Psychologists use of e-mail with clients: Some ethical considerations. *The Ohio Psychologist,* pp. 13–17. Retrieved from *http://kspope.com/ethics/email.php#copy.*

Dugas, M. J., & Ladouceur, R. (2000). Treatment of GAD: Targeting intolerance of uncertainty in two types of worry. *Behavior Modification, 24,* 635–657.

Durkheim, E. (1897). *Suicide.* Paris, France.

Ekman, P. (1999). Basic emotions. In T. Dalgleish & M. Power (Eds.). *Handbook of cognition and emotion.* Sussex, UK: Wiley.

Farmer, R. F., & Chapman, A. L. (2008). *Behavioral interventions in cognitive behavior therapy: Practical guidance for putting theory into action*. Washington, DC: American Psychological Association.

Farmer, R. F., & Chapman, A. L. (2016). *Behavioral interventions in cognitive behavior therapy: Practical guidance for putting theory into action* (2nd ed.). Washington, DC: American Psychological Association.

Fawcette, J., Scheftner, W., Fogg, L., Clark, D., Young, M., Hedeker, D., & Gibbons, R. (1990). Time-related predictors of suicide in major affective disorder. *American Journal of Psychiatry, 147*(9), 1189–1194.

Ferguson, K. E., & Christiansen, K. (2008). Shaping. In W. T. O'Donohue & J. E. Fisher (Eds.), *Cognitive behavior therapy: Applying empirically supported techniques in your practice* (2nd ed., pp. 493–501). Hoboken, NJ: Wiley.

Foa, E. B., & Rothbaum, B. O. (2001). *Treating the trauma of rape: Cognitive behavioral therapy for PTSD*. New York: Guilford Press.

Follette, V., Palm, K. M., & Pearson, A. N. (2006). Mindfulness and trauma: Implications for treatment. *Journal of Rational-Emotive and Cognitive-Behavior Therapy, 24*, 45–61.

Follette, W. C., & Callaghan, G. M. (1995). Do as I do, not as I say: A behavior-analytic approach to supervision. *Professional Psychology: Research and Practice, 26*, 413–421.

Fruzzetti, A. E., & Shenk, C. (2008). Fostering validating responses in families. *Social Work in Mental Health, 6*, 215–227.

Gailliot, M. T., & Baumeister, R. F. (2007). The physiology of willpower: Linking blood glucose to self-control. *Personality and Social Psychology Review, 11*, 303–327.

Goldfried, M. R., & Davison, G. R. (1976). *Clinical behavior therapy*. New York: Holt, Rinehart, & Winston.

Gross, J. J. (1998). The emerging field of emotion regulation: An integrative review. *Review of General Psychology, 2*(3), 271–299.

Gross, J. J. (Ed.). (2015). *Handbook of emotion regulation* (2nd ed.). New York: Guilford Press.

Hawton, K. K. E., Townsend, E., Arensman, E., Gunnell, D., Hazell, P., House, A., et al. (1999). Psychosocial and pharmacological treatments for deliberate self harm. *Cochrane Database of Systematic Reviews, Issue 4*, Article No. CD001754.

Immordino-Yang, M. H., Christodoulou, J. A., & Singh, V. (2012). Rest is not idleness: Implications of the brain's default mode for human development and education. *Perspectives on Psychological Science, 7*, 352–364.

Joiner, T. E. (2005). *Why people die by suicide*. Cambridge, MA: Harvard University Press.

Kazdin, A. E. (2012). *Behavior modification in applied settings* (7th ed.). Long Grove, IL: Waveland Press.

Koerner, K. (2012). *Doing dialectical behavior therapy: A practical guide.* New York: Guilford Press.

Kohlenberg, R. J., & Tsai, M. (1991). *Functional analytic psychotherapy: Creating intense and curative therapy relationships.* New York: Plenum Press.

Kurzban, R. (2010). Does the brain consume additional glucose during self-control tasks? *Evolutionary Psychology, 8,* 244–259.

Lannin, D. G., & Scott, N. A. (2014). Best practices for an online world. *American Psychological Association, 45,* 56–61.

LeDoux, J. (2002). *Synaptic self: How our brains become who we are.* New York: Viking.

Limbrunner, H. M., Ben-Porath, D. D., & Wisniewski, L. (2011, May). DBT telephone skills coaching with eating disordered clients: Who calls, for what reasons, and for how long? *Cognitive and Behavioral Practice, 18,* 186–195.

Linehan, M. M. (1993a). *Cognitive behavioral treatment of borderline personality disorder.* New York: Guilford Press.

Linehan, M. M. (1993b). *Skills training manual for treating borderline personality disorder.* New York: Guilford Press.

Linehan, M. M. (1997). Validation and psychotherapy. In A. C. Bohart & L. S. Greenberg (Eds.), *Empathy reconsidered: New directions in psychotherapy* (pp. 353–392). Washington, DC: American Psychological Association.

Linehan, M. M. (2014). *Linehan risk assessment and management protocol (LRAMP).* Seattle, WA: Behavioral Research and Therapy Clinics.

Linehan, M. M. (2015). *DBT skills training manual* (2nd ed.). New York: Guilford Press.

Linehan, M. M., Kanter, J., & Comtois, K. A. (1999). Dialectical behavior therapy for borderline personality disorder: Efficacy, specificity, and cost effectiveness. In D. S. Janowsky (Ed.), *Psychotherapy indications and outcomes* (pp. 93–118). Arlington, VA: American Psychiatric Association.

Locke, E. A., & Latham, G. P. (2002). Building a practically useful theory of goal setting and task motivation. *American Psychologist, 57,* 705–717.

Lunenberg, F. C. (2011). Goal-setting theory of motivation. *International Journal of Management, Business, and Administration, 15,* 1–5.

Lynch, T. R., Chapman, A. L., Rosenthal, M. Z., Kuo, J. K., & Linehan, M. M. (2006). Mechanisms of change in dialectical behavior therapy: Theoretical and empirical observations. *Journal of Clinical Psychology, 62,* 459–480.

Maldonado, J. R., & Garcia, R. (2016). Suicide risk assessment and management. In M. B. Riba (Ed.), *Clinical manual of emergency psychiatry* (2nd ed., pp. 33–68). Arlington, VA: American Psychiatry Association.

Manning, S. Y. (2011). Common errors made by therapists providing telephone consultation in dialectical behavior therapy. *Cognitive and Behavioural Practice, 18,* 178–185.

Mauss, I. B., & Tamir, M. (2013). Emotion goals: How their content, structure, and operation shape emotion regulation. In J. J. Gross (Ed.), *Handbook of emotion regulation* (2nd ed., pp. 361–375). New York: Guilford Press.

Martell, C. R., Dimidjian, S., & Herman-Dunn, R. (2010). *Behavioral activation for depression: A clinician's guide.* New York: Guilford Press.

Miller, A. J., Rathus, J., & Linehan, M. M. (2007). *Dialectical behavior therapy with suicidal adolescents.* New York: Guilford Press.

Miller, W. R., & Rollnick, S. (2002). *Motivational interviewing: Preparing people for change* (2nd ed.). New York: Guilford Press.

Miller, W. R., & Rollnick, S. (2012). *Motivational interviewing: Helping people change* (3rd ed.). New York: Guilford Press.

Nezu, A. M., & Nezu, C. M. (2012). Problem solving. In W. T. O'Donohue & J. E. Fisher (Eds.), *Cognitive behavior therapy: Core principles for practice* (pp. 159–182). New York: Wiley.

Nhat Hanh, T. (1996). *Being peace.* Berkeley, CA: Parallax Press.

Nock, M. K., & Prinstein, M. J. (2004). A functional approach to the assessment of self-mutilative behavior. *Journal of Consulting and Clinical Psychology, 72,* 885–890.

Ochsner, K. N., & Gross, J. J. (2014). The neural bases of emotion and emotion regulation: A valuation perspective. In J. J. Gross (Ed.), *Handbook of emotion regulation* (2nd ed., pp. 23–42). New York: Guilford Press.

Oliveira, P. N., & Rizvi, S. L. (in press). Phone coaching in dialectical behavior therapy: Frequency and relationship to client variables. *Cognitive Behaviour Therapy.*

Perlis, M. L., Jungquist, C., Smith, M. T., & Posner, D. (2006). *Cognitive behavioral treatment of insomnia: A session-by-session guide.* New York: Springer.

Persons, J. B., & Tompkins, M. A. (2007). Cognitive-behavioral case formulation. In T. D. Eells (Ed.), *Handbook of psychotherapy case formulation* (2nd ed., pp. 290–316). New York: Guilford Press.

Power, J., Smith, H. P., & Beaudette, J. N. (2016). Examining Nock and Prinstein's four-function model with offenders who self-injure. *Personality Disorders: Theory, Research, and Treatment, 7*(3), 309–314.

Pryor, K. (2012). *Don't shoot the dog: The new art of teaching and training.* Gloucestershire, UK: Ringpress Books.

Quinlan, R. J., & Quinlan, M. B. (2007). Evolutionary ecology of human pair-bonds: Cross-cultural tests of alternative hypotheses. *Cross-Cultural Research, 41*, 149–169.

Rathus, J. H., & Miller, A. L. (2014). *DBT skills manual for adolescents.* New York: Guilford Press.

Rosenthal, M. Z., & Kutlu, M. G. (2014). Translation of associative learning models into extinction reminders delivered via mobile phones during cue exposure interventions for substance use. *Psychology of Addictive Behaviors, 28*, 863–871.

Simon, R. I. (2012). Suicide risk assessment: Gateway to treatment and management. In R. E. Hales & R. I. Simon (Eds.), *The American Psychiatric Publishing textbook of suicide assessment and management* (pp. 3–28). Washington, DC: American Psychiatric Publications.

Steinburg, J. A., Steinburg, S. J., & Miller, A. L. (2011). Orienting adolescents and families to DBT telephone consultation: Principles, procedures, and pitfalls. *Cognitive and Behavioral Practice, 18*, 196–206.

Stoffers, J. M., Völlm, B. A., Rücker, G., Timmer, A., Huband, N., & Lieb, K. (2012). Psychological therapies for people with borderline personality disorder. *Cochrane Database of Systematic Reviews, 8*, Article No. CD005652.

Stolberg, R., & Bognar, B. (2009). Assessment of suicide risk. In J. Butcher (Ed.), *Oxford handbook of personality assessment* (pp. 501–526). New York: Oxford University Press.

Suvak, M. K., Litz, B. T., Sloan, D. M., Zanarini, M. C., Barrett, L. F., & Hofmann, S. G. (2011). Emotional granularity and borderline personality disorder. *Journal of Abnormal Psychology, 120*, 414–426.

Troister, T., D'Agata, M. T., & Holden, R. R. (2015). Suicide risk screening: Comparing the Beck Depression Inventory–II, Beck Hopelessness Scale, and Psychache Scale in undergraduates. *Psychological Assessment, 27*(4), 1500–1506.

Turner, B. J., Cobb, R. J., Gratz, K. L., & Chapman, A. L. (2016). The role of perceived interpersonal conflict and perceived social support in nonsuicidal self-injury in daily life. *Journal of Abnormal Psychology, 125*, 588–598.

Vaiva, G., Ducrocq, F., Meyer, P., Mathieu, D., Philippe, A., Libersa, C., & Goudemand, M. (2006). Effect of telephone contact on further suicide attempts in patients discharged from an emergency department: Randomised controlled study. *British Medical Journal, 332*, 1241–1245.

Zaki, L. F., Coifman, K. G., Rafaeli, E., Berenson, K. R., & Downey, G. (2013). Emotion differentiation as a protective factor against nonsuicidal self-injury in borderline personality disorder. *Behavior Therapy, 44*, 529–540.

Index

Note. *t* following a page numbers indicates a table.